DEDICATION

This book is dedicated to
courageous cancer patients
everywhere—and their
heroic caregivers.

There is hope.

STAY HEALTHY
DURING CHEMO

The Five Essential Steps

Mike Herbert, ND

with Joseph Dispenza, author of *Live Better Longer*

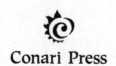

Conari Press

This edition first published in 2015 by Conari Press
an imprint of Red Wheel/Weiser, LLC
With offices at:
65 Parker Street, Suite 7
Newburyport, MA 01950
www.redwheelweiser.com
Sign up for our newsletter and special offers by going to www.redwheelweiser.com/
newsletter.

ISBN: 978-1-57324-675-0

Library of Congress Cataloging-in-Publication Data available upon request

Cover design by Jim Warner
Interior Design by landerro@mac.com

Printed in the United States of America
MG

10 9 8 7 6 5 4 3 2 1

Contents

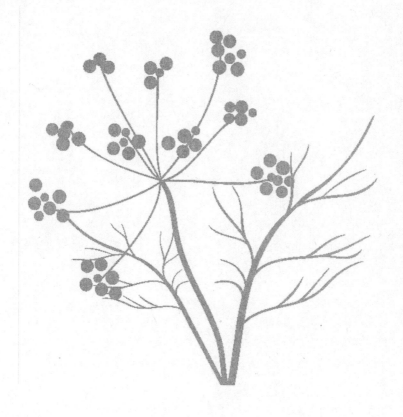

*Your present circumstances don't determine where
you can go; they merely determine where you start.*

Nido Qubein

Introduction

I am writing this book because when I faced a cancer crisis of my own, I could not find a book that would give me solid, reliable information fast enough.

Here is what happened. Out of the blue, my partner, who seemed to be enjoying perfect health up to then, was diagnosed with Stage IV Non-Hodgkin's Lymphoma. The disease was both virulent and aggressive, advancing daily throughout his body's lymphatic system and threatening to attack his internal organs.

After we got over the shock of an impending death sentence, we began to sort out what needed to be done. Both of us are confirmed natural healing advocates: I am a naturopathic doctor; he has written a book and scores of articles on alternative healing methods. By temperament and by training, we leaned toward seeking a cancer cure outside what is considered "conventional" medical procedure. But, mainly because of the cancer's rapid progress, we opted for traditional cancer treatment under the direction of a traditional oncologist.

We understood that choosing conventional treatment over some of the new alternative, complementary, and integrative approaches probably meant chemotherapy and radiation, maybe even surgery. These are the standard weapons used by allopathic (conventional Western) oncologists in the "war against cancer."

We also suspected that this arsenal of medical chemicals, especially in the case of chemotherapy, probably would be effective in attacking the cancer, but might not be helpful beyond that. I knew that chemotherapy is designed to kill cells in the body and will stop rapidly dividing cells from multiplying. That is what it will do. What chemo will not do is make a person healthy.

Overnight, I became both a full-time caregiver and nutritional researcher. I was highly motivated to find out how to help my partner stay alive. Because the cancer was advancing rapidly, I closed down my practice and put myself back in graduate school, with myself as the only student—as if I was working on another doctoral degree in naturopathy, this time with a specialization in staying healthy during chemotherapy.

So, we entered traditional cancer treatment—sometimes referred to as "the cancer treatment system"—but with our eyes wide open, looking for every opportunity to balance the destructive work of the chemo chemicals with constructive, life-boosting foods and supplements.

As my research progressed, I began introducing natural healing practices into my partner's personal anti-cancer program. The first order of business was to radically alter what he was eating. He had always been a careful eater, but the new situation called for a thorough scrutiny of the foods that had been his regular fare up to that point.

If the first big area of concern was what he was eating, the second, and just as important, was what he was taking—that is, supplements. My research was showing that the most highly trusted sources were endorsing the use of supplements during chemo, and in therapeutic doses, many times the daily dosage for a healthy person.

Six chemo treatments were prescribed by the doctor. They would be administered three weeks apart, allowing just enough time to recover from one session before undertaking the next. Again, because of the rapid spread of the disease, chemo would begin three days after the initial diagnosis.

Along with conventional treatment, which included not only the chemo drugs but also other pharmaceuticals for various side ailments before, during, and after the actual chemo days, we embarked on a strict regimen of a newly formulated diet, supplemented by vitamins, minerals, and herbs.

Detoxification was also a pressing issue because the chemo needed to leave the body as quickly as possible and take the dead cancer cells with it. I recommended that my partner take detox baths and coffee enemas, based on ideas put forth by highly respected natural healers who were using them with cancer patients.

Added to all this was an "exercise program"—a daily walk that began as a tentative stroll around the block and progressed to, in a couple of weeks, a nature hike of nearly two miles. Oddly, perhaps, I did not have to push this exercise on my partner. He did it on his own, at a time of the day when he had the energy, because, with the rich nutrients he was taking in, he felt up to walking and felt really good afterwards.

Several weeks went by, with some good days and some bad days—all bravely borne by my partner with anticipation of a bright light at the end of the dark tunnel of treatments. Meanwhile, I continued my investigation into how a person can stay healthy throughout conventional cancer therapy, using the power of nature and the body's own healing capabilities as allies.

During all this time, my partner suffered no nausea or vomiting, and rarely had diarrhea or constipation. There was no indigestion, no heartburn, no dehydration. These and other common side effects of chemo relating to food and drink seemed to be taken care of by a proper diet, one that allowed for optimum digestion and assimilation.

Sometimes, if he was up to it, we listened to informational tapes and watched videos together, comparing notes afterwards. In time, I had compiled several file folders bulging with data on the role of nutrition and supplementation in the treatment of cancer from the latest and most trustworthy sources. Study after study repeated the same encouraging message: keep a positive attitude, detox, eat right, supplement the diet, exercise.

A PET/CT scan after the third chemo treatment showed that no cancer was visible in my partner's body. Naturally, this was cause for optimism. But, as the oncologist kept reminding us, a scan only shows what is visible. To get at what was happening at the microscopic level, we would need more blood work, more probing, more examinations—and more chemotherapy.

But after the fifth round of chemo (of the prescribed six), the lab results were thought to be so good that a final round of the chemicals was deemed unnecessary. Choosing to stop chemo varied from the oncologist's original conservative prescription, but the chemo seemed to be doing more damage at this point than the cancer had done; although there were few physical side effects present, my partner's mental abilities seemed to be increasingly compromised. The oncologist agreed with us to shorten the chemotherapy treatment, or at least he did not insist on one more blast of chemo.

The nightmare that had begun in August was over and done with by Christmas. So far, the happy ending of this story is holding. The cancer, after almost a year, has not returned. And my partner has resumed his life fully, with mounting energy and enthusiasm to meet the bright future he had imagined during those dark days.

From a cancer patient, he has become a cancer survivor.

Every year in the United States alone, more than one and a half million people are handed the shocking cancer diagnosis that was given to my partner—that's the population of Phoenix or Philadelphia.

Imagine all those hundreds of thousands of people lined up to receive treatment for their cancers, hoping that they will receive the best treatment possible, that they will able to afford it, that the process of healing will be easy and not wrenching, and that they will come out the other side in good health and ready to pick up their lives where they left off before cancer.

Some eventually will call themselves cancer survivors, joining the twelve million in the U.S. Others will not.

Statistics on how many cancer patients will opt for conventional allopathic treatment, including chemotherapy, are hard to come by; numbers are difficult, maybe even impossible, to ascertain. Most sources that monitor the traffic in and out of hospitals and cancer clinics say that probably 90% of diagnosed patients will choose conventional treatment—surgery, chemotherapy, and radiation.

My experience with cancer—including chemotherapy and the other conventional treatments medical science has to combat it— left me with a burning desire to share the information I gathered with people who have been diagnosed with cancer.

Early on in my partner's life-or-death cancer journey, I realized I wanted to write a book that would outline a practical way to augment the healing process begun by the oncologist and other specialists. Their job is to eradicate cancer cells using highly toxic chemicals. The job of the cancer patient and the caregiver is to pick up the process where that leaves off by using sensible eating plans with supplements, natural herbal powders, juices, and teas, combined with detoxifications and exercise—all designed to build up the immune system, help lessen the debilitating side effects of chemotherapy, keep the cancer patient healthy and more energetic during treatment, and speed up the healing process.

I am writing this book to tell cancer patients they can heal faster and better during their time in conventional treatment. This can be done by turning to the body's own self-correcting, self-healing capability for assistance.

The program I am setting out here starts with the idea that our bodies are potent healing machines and that well-being is our normal, natural state. Even under the assault of the toxic chemicals that make up chemotherapy—the more toxic the better, to destroy cancer cells—there is a great deal that can be done to help mitigate their side effects and to promote healing by activating and fueling the body's immune system, allowing it to operate as a powerful healing engine. Remember that even at the time of diagnosis, we have more healthy cells than cancer cells in our body.

Let me say here that what follows comes from my personal experience as a doctor of naturopathy and a caregiver to my partner and from the evidence of clients who come to me for help. It is not a scientific study or a laboratory tested procedure. I designed this program from my knowledge of natural medicine, learned over more than a decade of treating clients with various body imbalances.

This book admittedly presents a one-size-fits-all approach, even though it is important to acknowledge that every person and every cancer is different. Women with cancer are different from men with cancer; children with cancer are different from adults with cancer; people with lung cancer are different from people with stomach cancer. As humans, however, we share a common chemistry and that has been my guide in assembling a support plan that will benefit anyone seeking to stay healthy during chemotherapy and those returning to normal life...cancer-free.

If you are a cancer patient or a caregiver, I send you personal wishes for health, well-being, and a future filled with passion and joy. There is hope!

Please note that the information here is not meant to replace any therapy for cancer set out by a primary health provider. Before undertaking any of the suggestions I put forth in this book, a cancer patient and caregiver should check with the oncologist or other medical professional who is mainly responsible for treatment.

A Note about Our Website

All the information I assembled about staying healthy while undergoing chemotherapy could not fit in this book, so my team and I expanded the essential material you will find here into a website.

On the site you will see more recipes, charts that can be printed out for posting around the kitchen, sources for the highest quality supplements, educational articles, free downloads, and more.

The new field of staying healthy during cancer treatment is changing rapidly, with new research appearing virtually every day. I encourage you to visit our website frequently for up-to-the-minute information and inspiration.

stayhealthyduringchemo.com

PART ONE

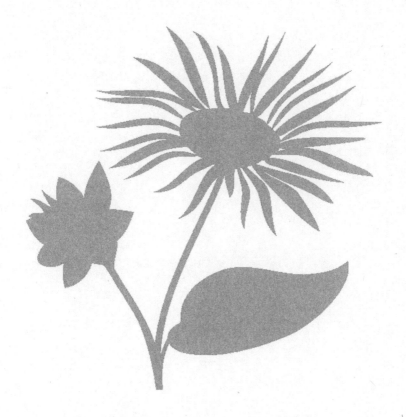

*Chemotherapy
Is Only Part of the
Healing Process*

PART ONE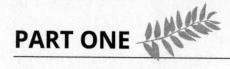

Chemotherapy Is Only Part of the Healing Process

> The doctor of the future will give no medication, but will interest his patients in the care of the human frame, diet, and in the cause and prevention of disease.
>
> *Thomas A. Edison*

Cancer and Chemo

• In recent years, according to the American Cancer Society's Global Cancer Facts & Figures, over 12 million new cancer cases were diagnosed each year and 7.6 million cancer deaths—about 20,000 cancer deaths a day—occurred worldwide.

• Around 150 people are diagnosed with cancer every hour in the United States. Over a year, that amounts to almost 1.6 million people in the United States alone.

• One out of every four Americans is diagnosed with cancer each year. This year about 564,800 Americans are expected to die of cancer—more than 1,500 people a day, day after day, week after week.

• Cancer is the second leading cause of death in the United States, exceeded only by heart disease.

• One of every four deaths in the United States is from cancer.

- Cancer is expensive: the health care industry in the United States—which includes doctors, hospitals and clinics, pharmaceutical companies, manufacturers of medical technology, insurance companies, and so on—comprises around 10% of the Gross Domestic Product (GDP), or around $1.5 trillion in 2011.

- Of the million and a half plus American people with cancer, the vast majority opts for treatment by conventional medicine…and at least 75% receives chemotherapy as part of the routine method for dealing with the disease.

- Chemotherapy, either by itself or in conjunction with radiation and surgery, has become the standard treatment for most cancers in conventional medical practice.

We Can't Rely on Chemo Alone

Many cancer patients seem to have attached themselves to the idea that chemotherapy solves all the problems that cancer poses. They believe that between chemo and radiation treatments, everything that can be done to destroy the cancer and bring the patient back to good health is automatically being done.

Call it the antibiotic mind-set. When we take antibiotics, we assume that they are combating an infection in the body brought on by bacteria or fungi or parasites, and we don't need to do anything else to push the process of infection-fighting further. The antibiotics are taking care of everything.

Let me say immediately that chemotherapy is not the same as antibiotic or antibacterial therapy. The medications are quite different and so are the processes of how they work. But the mind-set of "let medicine do the work while I just sit back and wait" is the same with chemo as it is with antibiotics for many people.

Cancer patients who are not suffering from a cancer related to the digestive process—such as stomach, pancreatic or colon cancer—are usually allowed an "unrestricted diet" by their oncologists. For instance, my partner who was diagnosed with lymphoma needed to be hospitalized for his first round of chemotherapy because he had a history of hepatitis-B and his doctor did not want to risk a flare-up of that disease during the chemo treatments. Chemo would suppress the immune system, leaving the door open for other diseases to come out of hiding. So the first chemo cocktail was administered as a round-the-clock drip over five days.

All during that week in the hospital, since his diet was officially "unrestricted," he was served the same kinds of food available to anyone eating in the cafeteria-style restaurant down the street. A typical dinner was Salisbury steak with mashed potatoes and gravy, a salad with ranch dressing, bread roll and butter, a glass of milk, a cup of coffee, and for dessert, a generous slice of chocolate cake.

During the time that chemo was being administered—his entire stay in the hospital—he was not allowed supplements of any kind, because of the concern that vitamins, minerals, and amino acids might have interfered with the intended effects of chemotherapy, and in some cases might have actually caused dangerous chemical reactions in the body. This, in spite of the fact that most foods naturally contain vitamins, minerals, and amino acids.

So my partner was left with chemo and an "unrestricted diet," which is to say that there was precious little to rely on for healing beyond chemotherapy and a business-as-usual eating plan.

Once out of the hospital, he was put on a regular schedule of chemotherapy treatments every three weeks. His prescription was for five day-long treatments following the week-long drip in the hospital—making six rounds of chemo over eighteen weeks, a period of five months, six counting follow-up blood work and PET scans.

All during that critical half-year period, he was left in chemo treatment only with the usual unrestricted diet directive and the admonition to avoid all supplements on the chemo days. Nothing was said about adding or subtracting foods and beverages from his diet or engaging in some gentle exercise such as walking or yoga, or anything else beyond getting chemo and, as best he could, recovering from one round in time to take another round.

Left with this regimen for healing, which is no regimen at all, a cancer patient can look forward to weeks and months of feeling bad from the side effects of chemotherapy as the body processes and then finally eliminates the toxic chemicals along with the dead cancer cells. Meanwhile, the body is left in such a weakened state that the patient often becomes a professional sick person, open to all kinds of lesser diseases that a compromised immune system lets in.

Something is missing. There must be a way for a cancer patient to withstand the forceful work of chemo in the body and feel good at the same time. There must be a way to speed up the process of healing from cancer and enjoy high energy and a sense of well-being while the healing is taking its course.

There is a way, of course, and it is nature's way.

What Chemo Is Designed to Do

To understand more about what really goes on in chemo treatment, it is important to know what chemotherapy is designed to do. Chemotherapy treats cancer with an antineoplastic drug or several antineoplastic drugs in combination. "Antineoplastic" means that a drug acts to prevent, inhibit, or stop (anti) the development of a tumor (neoplasm).

The task of chemotherapy chemicals is to kill rapidly dividing malignant cells in the body. Cancer cells divide and multiply at a rapid rate, causing a breakdown in bodily systems. Chemotherapy kills those cells, and along with them the reproducing cells of normal tissues. The chemicals can be given through a vein, which is the usual way of getting them into the body, or injected into a body cavity. Sometimes one or more of the chemicals are given orally in pill form.

When chemo descends to do fatal damage to malignant cells and stop the disease from spreading, it also damages normal cells. And when that happens, unwanted side effects appear. Since chemo cannot tell the difference between a cancer cell and a healthy cell, it attacks both the rapidly growing cancer cells and other fast-growing cells, such as hair and blood cells.

A cancer patient already knows most of this, because it is part of the experience of living with chemo treatment. Naturally, an oncologist tries to find a delicate balance between destroying the malignant cells to control the disease and leaving the normal cells alone, so that there are as few negative side effects as possible.

So, chemo is designed to kill. There is some interesting history behind this language of killing, destroying, and attacking. The chemical treatment of cancer goes back to the world wars of the past century and the development of weaponry.

During World War I, one of the weapons deployed was chlorine gas, which was used as early as 1915. Another was mustard gas. So devastating were the effects of these and other chemical gases—killing, in many cases, both sides in a battle—that their use in warfare was banned. But it was found that mustard gas was a powerful suppressor of hematopoiesis, or blood production. Based on those findings, medical scientists began to study how chemicals derived from nitrogen mustards might arrest the growth of cancer cells.

In 1942, during World War II, an accident exposed several hundred people to mustard gas in the Italian town of Bari. Those who survived were discovered to have very low white blood cell counts. After the war, researchers experimented with using chemicals to fight cancer, starting with mustine, developed from nitrogen mustards.

The first chemotherapy drugs were born in warfare and have never lost their bellicose expression. In the 1970s and 1980s, when cancer began to emerge as "the emperor of all diseases," as one recent book calls it, cancer patients were encouraged to engage in noble combat with the disease, imagining healthy cells in the body doing battle against cancer cells—and winning.

Allusions to chemotherapy's wartime past are also evident in how we frame the treatment of "aggressive" cancers that "advance" rapidly and therefore must be killed, destroyed, eradicated, wiped out, exterminated. When the National Cancer Act of 1971 was announced, it was immediately named "the War on Cancer" by the media. Other efforts to support cancer research are routinely referred to in warlike terms. Obituaries report that a person "lost his battle against cancer."

These warlike allusions attached to chemotherapy are entirely appropriate, since chemo does indeed kill—and, as I have said before, when it does, it destroys healthy cells along with cancerous ones. The challenge for cancer patients and caregivers is to allow chemo to do its destructive work on malignant cells, while at the same time trying to stay healthy enough to withstand the onslaught (another warfare term) of the necessarily lethal chemicals.

Since 1971, when President Richard Nixon declared war on cancer, the United States has spent $2 trillion on conventional cancer treatment and research, but it is a war we appear to have lost. Mortality rates are about the same as they were in 1950. To give a further warlike perspective, more Americans will die of cancer in the next fourteen months than have died from all the wars that the United States has fought combined.

Even though chemotherapy has its roots in war, a cancer patient does not have to become attached to the battle images that arise when discussing treatment. In fact, I think it is best not to envision a war raging inside the body of a cancer patient; better to see it as a healing process that is taking its course to well-being.

What Chemo Will Not Do

Chemotherapy is designed to kill cells in the body and, by accomplishing that, will stop rapidly dividing cells from multiplying. That is what it will do. What chemo will not do is make a person healthy.

The mission of chemo is a quick and thorough seek out, find, and destroy operation, to call upon more warlike terms. The rest is about staying healthy during chemo treatment and returning to vibrant well-being after the toxic chemicals and the residue from dead cancer cells have passed out of the body.

It is important to remember that chemotherapy will not heal the body, since it is not designed to do that. What chemotherapy will do is destroy cells. The idea here is that once cancer cells are attacked and removed, the body can then take over and heal itself.

When cancer cells are no longer viable and cease to divide and multiply, they are flushed out of the body as waste material. At that point the environment in the body is changed from a functioning system compromised by a spreading cancer to a system that promotes the body's well-being. Changing the environment creates the healing scenario.

I mention this here, because there is often a misunderstanding among cancer patients that chemotherapy actually does the healing work involved in recovering from cancer. It does not heal, but it sets the scene for healing by getting rid of the offending aberrant cells. Tumors will go away or be reduced, and other symptoms brought on by the cancer will vanish, hopefully, including pain, bodily discharges, and so on. Returning to good health, though, is another issue entirely.

Chemotherapy will not make a cancer patient well; it will, however, and under the best of circumstances, destroy the cancer that is preventing wellness. In other words, chemo will not produce the solution, but it will help to take away the problem. That is something enormous, of course, and needs to be acknowledged and respected. To keep with the warlike metaphors that chemo has suggested since its creation, it is powerful ammunition for a seek-and-destroy medical mission.

Another thing that chemotherapy will not accomplish has to do with the immune system. Chemo is so potent, as I've said before, that it weakens the body's own means of protecting itself, which is why so many people on chemo will come down with colds or the flu or worse on their way to being healed from cancer.

Let's remember that chemotherapy is not intended to, and therefore will not, promote the body's self-healing mechanism directly, although it does so indirectly by helping change the environment in which the cancer is thriving. A cancer patient's immune system, after it is compromised by the attacks on cancerous cells, will rise and fall with no help from chemo itself. To protect and enhance immunity, much will depend on what is done outside of the chemo clinic.

Chemo's Negative Side Effects

The positive effect of chemotherapy, in the best of circumstances, is the killing of cancer cells in the body of a cancer patient. But, as we all know, along with the good comes the bad. The distress accompanying chemotherapy is for some almost as difficult to endure as the cancer itself.

Invariably, a person who has been diagnosed with cancer will receive, along with a schedule of chemotherapy treatments (assuming chemo has been prescribed), a list of the precise drugs that will be used and their "possible" side effects. As if the catalog of the drugs and their descriptions is daunting enough, the litany of side effects is scary indeed.

The following are the most common side effects of chemotherapy, depending on the type of cancer, the type of chemo drugs administered, and their dosages. Not every cancer patient will experience all of the side effects, but most will experience at least some of them.

Immune system depression is the first, most obvious, and most dangerous. The immune system is suppressed to the point where the body can be prey to illness and infections that would ordinarily be quite harmless. This is why doctors will tell chemo patients to avoid crowds, where they might come into contact with contagious potentially dangerous bacteria and viruses. For a healthy person to be in a room with someone who has a cold is no problem; for the chemo patient, it could mean days or weeks suffering the contracted cold—sometimes it might even result in a hospital stay.

Fatigue is the result of fighting both the cancer and the chemo. It is always mentioned in the literature of what to expect from chemotherapy treatment. In some cases, anemia will be detected and drugs will be prescribed to address it. Most cancer patients can be spotted for their tired and haggard looks, slow movements, and cloudy thinking—all of which are symptoms of fatigue. Most of the fatigue is due directly to the accumulation of toxins in the liver.

Hair loss occurs almost immediately after the first chemo treatment. It happens because the chemotherapy drugs go after all rapidly dividing cells, and hair follicles are among the fastest-growing cells in the body. This is a physical effect that has tremendous emotional and psychological counterparts. Almost all cancer patients report the shock they felt at first seeing all their hair gone, straining to recognize the person in the mirror.

Damage to other parts of the body is also a potential side effect of chemotherapy. An oncologist will be on the lookout for breakdowns in areas of the body that may not be contaminated with cancer, but are the result of the powerful work of the chemo. These areas include, but are not confined to, the heart, the liver, the kidneys, the inner ear (manifesting as imbalance), and the brain.

Chemo brain. On the subject of the brain, cancer patients on chemo will almost universally report fogginess in thinking, forgetting things, an inability to come up with the right word, and so on. These lapses are more than the ordinary brain stops-and-starts that are part of virtually everyone's experience. For a person receiving chemo treatments, this is part of the process and can be emotionally painful and perilous, especially when important prescribed medications are forgotten.

Nausea and vomiting are so common among those on chemo that they are usually the first things an oncologist will mention to a patient. Other gastrointestinal problems, including diarrhea and constipation, go with the territory. Sometimes, these become issues of huge proportions, causing rapid weight loss or weight gain, chronic indigestion and heartburn, malnutrition, dehydration, and other complications associated with the gastrointestinal system.

The Other Part of Healing

As we have seen, chemotherapy is only a part of the healing scenario for a cancer patient. Certainly, it is an essential element for those who have chosen a conventional route to treat cancer. But, while chemo is a powerful attacker of cancer cells, it is not a cure-all for the disease.

The other part of healing from cancer is the challenge of staying healthy through the span of chemo treatments and remaining in good health after those treatments have run their course. It is no small challenge for the cancer patient, particularly in the run-down physical and emotional state left in the wake of the chemo drugs.

What is required to stay healthy is, in the first place, a willingness to engage in the healing process. Many cancer patients simply turn their healing program over to their oncologist and assume that the doctor will take care of everything necessary to return to good health. This is the doctor-as-garage-mechanic attitude: I take my body into the shop, the doctor fixes it, and I go home. It is a mistake that could be fatal—and sometimes is literally that for thousands of people with cancer.

In our culture, we might even say that the role of the doctor has less to do with creating good health than in managing disease. We ask an oncologist to treat our cancer, but that does not automatically mean that we are asking the doctor to restore us to vibrant well-being. In fact, with our medical system of disease management (as opposed to health fostering), it actually would be presumptuous of us to expect more of our physicians than what they offer. And what they offer is considerable, if we want to eradicate cancer from the body.

Engaging the process of healing means that we do not rely on doctors alone to give us good health. They do their part by trying sincerely to rid the body of a rapidly growing disease. The rest is up to the cancer patient. This is not an easy thing to commit to, but unless one does, there can be no real healing.

So, what does the cancer patient do to fill in the blanks left by a system that goes only as far as managing the disease—in this case, destroying cancer and removing it from the body?

- First, as I said earlier, is to decide to undertake one's own healing and not assume that a doctor or a nurse or a hospital staff member is going to do it; they won't because that is not what they do, it's not their job.

- Next is to try to get as much information as possible—good, reliable, authoritative information—to form a structure for a healing program. I am writing this book to help provide just that.

- Finally, a cancer patient will need to have a dedicated caregiver. This is so important that I am going to say more about it in a separate section that follows. All the good resolutions a person with cancer makes will come to naught without the help of someone who is physically and mentally on top of things.

The All-Important Caregiver

There is such a thing as "chemo brain," or "chemo head." Do a search on the Internet for these terms and thousands of sites will come up. Although this has been a problem for cancer patients since the dawn of chemotherapy, the issue has only recently been named. It is now recognized as something that happens to most patients in chemo treatment, and it is being studied to see how it might be dealt with medically.

I mentioned this above as one of the side effects of chemo-therapy. But it bears repeating in discussing the role of the care-giver. There is a wide range of estimates of how many people get chemo brain. Some experts tell us that, among people who receive chemo, between 15% and 70% will experience brain symptoms. Others put the upper limit of the range at 50%. Working with these numbers, the risk of chemo brain can be higher than 1 out of 2 or as low as 1 in 6.

According to the American Cancer Society, patients with chemo brain experience these symptoms:

- They forget things that they usually have no trouble recalling (memory lapses).

- They have trouble concentrating (can't focus on what they're doing, have a short attention span, may "space out").

- They will have trouble remembering details like names, dates, and sometimes larger events.

- There will be problems in multi-tasking, such as answering the phone while cooking, without losing track of one task (they are less able to do more than one thing at a time).

- They take longer to finish things (disorganized, slower at think-ing and processing).

- There will be problems remembering common words (unable to find the right words to finish a sentence).

The American Cancer Society goes on to say that:

"For most people, chemo brain effects happen quickly and only last a short time. Others have long-term mental changes. Usually the changes that patients notice are very subtle, and others around them may not even notice any changes at all. Still, the people who are having problems are well aware of the differences in their thinking. Many people do not tell their cancer care team about this problem until it affects their everyday life."

Many cancer patients are embarrassed about chemo brain and try to cover up their forgetfulness and fuzzy thinking. At the heart of the matter is how the condition, temporary or not, can affect a patient's care. All too often, chemo brain will interfere with treatment because a patient forgets to take medications or gets confused about other aspects of treatment, including missing doctor appointments.

The need for a caregiver should be obvious, given the prevalence of chemo brain. Even a cancer patient who is not plagued with the extremes of this problem will have trouble remembering everything that has to be done during treatment, including the number and timing of medications, meetings with the oncologist and other medical specialists, getting scans and blood tests, fasting before certain examinations, filling prescriptions, and so on.

I believe that caregivers are a special breed of people, and their work is a spiritual practice. If a cancer patient is lucky, there will be a life-partner, family member, or friend who will be there to help. Assistance is necessary not only for the strictly medical reasons I mentioned, but also to keep track of the health-building program that augments chemotherapy. Without a trusted helper working side-by-side with the cancer patient, the healing journey will be long, arduous, and perilous. With the caregiver sharing the responsibility for recovery, that journey becomes a shared experience of combined intention, a comfort for each, and even a joy.

Adopting a Healing Lifestyle

And finally, before outlining the details of the program I have put together to help cancer patients and their caregivers, let me say something about a healthy lifestyle.

Cancer, like all life-threatening diseases, can be a wake-up call to live in a different way. Medical issues do not appear out of nowhere, even though they may seem to ambush and descend upon us at the least likely moment. The truth is we do much to bring about ill health on ourselves, whether consciously or unconsciously. The origins of cancer are myriad and often deeply mysterious, for the most part. But surely our lifestyle has much to do with our health and well-being.

When a diagnosis comes, many cancer patients will automatically go into denial about taking responsibility for their sickness. For some, the sentence of cancer—and it might even be a death sentence—has been levied upon them for no reason at all by an angry or capricious God, universe, force, or whatever. They see themselves as innocent victims of the disease, faultless for having contracted it.

More than 200 scientists under the auspices of the World Cancer Research Fund (WCRF) took five years to produce the most authoritative report we have on the role played by food, drink, obesity, and exercise in causing cancer. Their conclusion was that a third of cancers worldwide are caused by lifestyle choices—the quality of what we eat and how much or how little we exercise.

A study of nearly 45,000 sets of twins found that environment and lifestyle were stronger predictors than genetic factors when determining who might get prostate, colorectal and breast cancer.

A recent Cancer Research UK report found that 40% of cancers can be blamed on personal lifestyle. The study says that more than 100,000 cancers in Britain each year are caused by smoking, unhealthy diet (a lack of fruit and vegetables), misuse of alcohol, and being overweight.

In many cases, a cancer patient is indeed blameless in having created the situation that ended with a diseased body. Accidents, issues of heredity, or just being in the wrong place at the wrong time can cause cancer, notwithstanding precautions taken or preventions exercised. But, that said, we need to take responsibility for what we eat, drink, smoke, how we move and, in general, how we live our lives.

Admitting our own part in illness is the first step toward adopting a healthy lifestyle, one that is grounded in eating whole foods, drinking vitality-enhancing beverages, exercising regularly, and refraining from bad habits such as smoking, overworking, not getting enough sleep.

Working through this program requires a commitment to a healthy way of living. That can be done by owning up to how we have taken care of ourselves in the past and resolving to take better care now and in the future.

What follows is a practical way to augment the healing process begun by the oncologist and other specialists. Their job is to eradicate cancer cells using highly toxic chemicals. The job of the cancer patient and the caregiver is to pick up the process where that leaves off, using sensible eating plans, supplements, natural herbal powders, juices, and teas combined with detoxifications and exercise—all designed to build up the immune system, help lessen the debilitating side effects of chemotherapy, keep the cancer patient healthy and more energetic during treatment, and speed up the healing process.

My guide throughout is to work hand-in-hand with nature and with the body's own healing powers. This program is for anyone who has been diagnosed as having cancer, regardless of gender, type of cancer, or the stage of the disease.

As I have said before, anyone wanting to embark on this parallel journey of natural healing will need to check with the oncologist who prescribed chemotherapy. You may want to ask how much nutritional training the oncologist in charge of your healing has had. Knowing that can help you understand where the doctor's recommendations about diet and supplementation originate.

This is not only the usual disclaimer made in all matters pertaining to health and healing, it is also a caution for the cancer patient to be aware that certain foods or vitamins, minerals, or other supplements may counteract the effectiveness of the medical treatment. These cases are rare, but they can happen. Please practice due diligence and go the extra step to ensure that this program for healing is entirely successful.

PART TWO

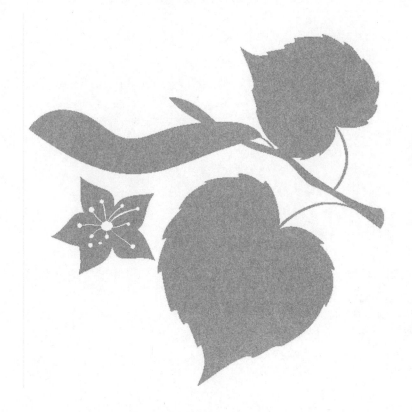

*The 5-Step
Chemotherapy Diet
Program*

PART TWO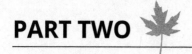

The 5-Step Chemotherapy Diet Program

> We must turn to nature itself, to the observations of the
> body in health and in disease to learn the truth.
>
> *Hippocrates*

The Chemotherapy Diet

Here is a quick summary of the 5-step program I developed for cancer patients and their caregivers. I will go through each step and say why it is important. Then, the rest of this section will be devoted to the actual nuts-and-bolts of the diet—what to do, how to do it, when, and why.

- **Step 1:** Change your thinking and develop an attitude focused on healing

- **Step 2:** Detoxify to promote healing from the inside out

- **Step 3:** Eat the best foods to create a healing chemistry in your body

- **Step 4:** Supplement your diet correctly to support the healing momentum

- **Step 5:** Exercise and rest to speed the healing process.

Let me explain that I am laying these steps out this way, each building on the one before it, as a way of fully engaging in the process of staying healthy during chemotherapy. Reading through these steps, you may be tempted to go directly to the list of foods to enjoy or avoid and begin there, skipping the detox step. Or you may want to start by taking supplements, leaving behind the all-important dietary guidelines. But if you look closely at each step, you will see that there is logic to the progression. If the program is followed as it is set out, you should have excellent results—staying healthy during treatment and beyond.

Step 1: Change Your Thinking and Develop an Attitude Focused on Healing

Healing is a matter of time, but it is sometimes also a matter of opportunity.

Hippocrates

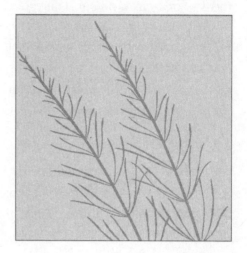

This step comes first, because an attitude that focuses on vibrant well-being creates the mental and emotional framework for the entire healing process. Expecting a successful outcome of the chemotherapy experience, and what you are adding to it with this program, will help to bring about that result.

It goes without saying that the reverse is also true. Cancer patients who begin a healing journey weighted down with fear, anxiety, self-pity, and an expectation of failure will find the road to wellness rocky, slippery, and barely navigable. Focus on failure, in other words, and you are bound to fail; focus on success, and you must surely succeed.

A re-identification is required here from cancer "victim" to cancer "victor"—and the body from diseased organism to healing machine.

Welcome to a new way of thinking about your relationship to cancer and chemotherapy! Whereas before you may have been dwelling on the "why me, why now?" part of being a cancer patient, the time has come to get positive and begin to develop an attitude focused on healing—your healing.

This really is the first step on the path of healing, no matter how you look at it. Diet, supplements, exercise—anything else you do for yourself to stay healthy during chemo—will be tougher and seem more scattered without this positive framework for the healing process.

I strongly urge you to engage these practices at the outset of the program, and to keep them going throughout. If you don't feel up to handling all of the suggestions below, try at least some of them. Tremendous benefits can be derived from "getting your head on straight" about who you are (not a victim, but a person on a healing journey) and where you are (exactly in the right place) in the process of getting and staying well.

Use Daily Affirmations

Affirmations are highly effective ways to turn around your thinking, and from there to turn around behavior. They have been used for centuries in one way or another to support goals and aspirations.

Affirmations are statements that you make to yourself, about yourself. You say them aloud and keep printed copies of them around (on your computer monitor, for instance) where you can see them and repeat them often during the day.

It's best to come up with an affirmation or two that you adopt as your own. Avoid using negative words, such as "no" or "not"—it is better to say "I am healthy" than to say "I do not have cancer."

Here are some suggestions:

• I am healthier with each new day.

• My body heals quickly and easily.

• I am healthy in every cell of my body.

• My body is a healing machine.

And before a nap or bedtime:

• Even when I am asleep, my body is healing itself.

Journal Your Feelings

Emotions are apt to run rampant during cancer treatment. You may find that you are happy one minute, depressed the next, on an ever-changing see-saw.

To bring some balance into the life of the emotions, and to release negative ones that might be weighing you down, consider keeping a journal of your feelings. It is as simple and getting a notebook, titling it "My Journal of Feelings," and writing in it once a day or several times a day, or whenever something comes up that you want to express.

There is no special way of doing this, except that the entries should always start with, "I am feeling...."

You may want to make your journal public. To do that, there is no better way than to blog on the Internet. Starting and maintaining a blog is not difficult; for some, it is a good way to both release emotions and share the experience of treatment.

Here are some emotions that may surface when you are doing this practice:

- Anger   • Gratitude

- Confusion   • Joy

- Fear   • Resentment

- Forgiveness   • Self-pity

Spruce Up Your Environment

Just because you are in treatment it doesn't mean you need to live in an environment that says "professional sick person." As part of the healing process, I encourage you to spruce up your surroundings, making them bright, airy, clean, and uncluttered.

Your outer world mirrors your inner world. If you are indeed on a journey of healing, it makes sense that the rooms where you are spending your time reflect the positive outlook you have adopted.

Here are a few ideas to make this a reality:

• Ask your caregiver and friends to bring you some fresh flowers every few days

• Make sure your bedroom is spotlessly clean and organized

• Unclutter—even if it means giving away a few things that may have lost their meaning for you

• Bring nature into your surroundings, whether through a small plant or photos of beautiful natural settings, or a bowl of water onto which you float some flower blossoms..

Dress Up

This goes hand-in-hand with the previous suggestion, but gets more personal. If you are spending a lot of time around the house—and close to the bed or couch, probably—there is something about freshening up and dressing up that is positively life-affirming.

Try to make time at least twice a week to dress up and go out, whether to an art gallery, a mall, a café, a park, or a movie—anywhere people congregate and pass by. This has a way of making us feel more "normal" than just sitting at home with a book or the TV.

Dressing up and going people-watching is good for the soul as well as for the body. When you get back to home-base, you may feel bushed, but will also feel fulfilled.

Stay Positive

Finally, wrap everything you do and say in a positive frame. Decide not to complain, but to be grateful for the good that is unfolding in your healing process. The more you concentrate on the positive aspects of your journey through chemo, the greater chance you have to heal faster and better.

Let "the glass is half-full" (not half-empty) be your mantra.

Step 2: Detoxify to Promote Healing from the Inside Out

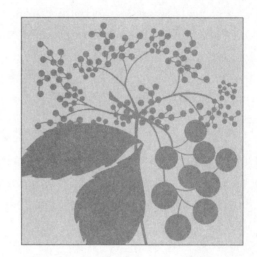

The wound is the place where the Light enters you.

Rumi

Once the new mental and emotional framework has been set in place, the practical work of getting healthy begins. And it all starts with cleaning the body of both the chemo drugs and the dead cancer cells they destroyed.

Detoxification is a kind of purification rite that acts as a gateway for all the marvelous life-enhancing changes that will take place during the healing process. It is vitally important that the toxic residue from cancer cells left behind by chemotherapy exits the body as quickly as possible. This step is about pushing the wastes of chemo out so they don't keep circulating in the body, endangering the precious environment of the immune system.

Toxins leave the body in several ways. Here we will be concentrating on detoxification through the digestive system, the skin (the body's largest organ), and the liver and bladder.

Cancer cells that are killed off by chemotherapy, the chemo chemicals themselves, and other toxins left behind on the chemo battlefield circulate in the body until they are processed and expelled by the eliminative organs—the liver, kidneys, bladder, lungs, lymphatic system, colon, blood, and the largest of our organs, the skin.

The sooner the accumulated toxins leave the body, the better! In this step, I am setting out two scientifically grounded detoxification regimes that are easy to do and require little preparation or special materials. They will help you to feel better faster.

External: Therapeutic Bathing

These four therapeutic baths come from the work of Dr. Hazel Parcells (1889-1996), a pioneer in the field of nutrition and holistic healing; if you do the math on her dates, you will see that she lived into her 107th year. You can also find them in *Live Better Longer,* the book about Dr. Parcells and her methods of natural healing.

I recommend that you take all four baths—one at a time, of course—over a two-week period. Then begin the round again, separating baths by a few days.

Therapeutic bathing is another way of cleansing, and therefore of healing. Our skin is an organ of our bodies—the largest organ. Sixty-five percent of body cleansing is accomplished through our skin.

The Underlying Scientific Principle

The Parcells therapeutic baths are based on the chemical principle "the weak will draw from the strong." The hot water bathing solution draws toxins out of the body to the surface of the skin. Then, as the water cools, the toxins are pulled from the surface of the skin by the change in temperature and go into the water. The purification is brought about by the simple principle of nature that the weak (cool water) energy draws from the strong (body heated by the hot water).

It is important to remain in the bath until the water cools in order to receive the full effect of these detoxifying therapeutic baths. Adding cold water to speed up the cooling of the bath water will change the chemistry of the bath, so that is not advised.

After leaving the tub, it is best to lie down covered with a blanket and allow your body to perspire freely, releasing more of the toxic build-up from the treatment process.

A general caution: depending where you are in chemo treatment, you may have to adjust the timing of these baths to make them tolerable to your system. You may find it uncomfortable and unpleasant to stay in the baths for more than ten or fifteen minutes. In that case, it is best to work up to a full therapeutic bath over several bathing sessions.

NOTE: it is not advisable to do a therapeutic bath on the day of chemo treatment or on the days before and after chemo.

The Four Parcells Therapeutic Bathing Formulas

Formula 1

When to Do It: This formula is especially good after any kind of scan. PET Scans and CAT Scans, for instance, will greatly increase levels of radiation in our bodies. Even simple dental X-rays will leave deposits in the body that will interfere with healthy functioning.

How to Do It: Dissolve 1 pound of sea salt or rock salt and 1 pound of baking soda in a tub of water as hot as can be tolerated. Stay in the bath until the water has cooled, at least 45 minutes. Do not shower for at least eight hours following the bath.

Formula 2

When to Do It: If you have been exposed to heavy metals, such as aluminum, or to carbon monoxide or unburned carbons, pesticide sprays, or deterrents. Cooking with aluminum will bring on symptoms. Eating foods that have not been cleaned of pesticides can lead to accumulations of pesticides in the cells.

This formula is excellent for a general detox, particularly if you are experiencing a general feeling of being "out of sorts," decreased energy, upper respiratory discomfort, a shortness of breath, light-headedness, or impaired balance.

How to Do It: Add 1 cup of Clorox brand bleach (non-scented) to a tub of water as hot as can be tolerated. Stay in the bath until the water has cooled, at least 45 minutes. Do not shower for at least eight hours following the bath.

Note: When people read a recommendation like the one above—that they should actually allow bleach to touch their skin—their eyebrows go up. Rest assured, the amount of bleach recommended here, in a solution of this much water, cannot hurt you. In fact, it can and will remove toxins with utmost effectiveness because it is a powerful oxygenator. Hospitals use bleach to disinfect because it removes viruses, germs, and bacteria. In a bath, its purpose is to disinfect the body, removing pesticides, metals, and carbon monoxide, among other toxins.

Be sensible, of course—don't use more bleach than is recommended. But do be adventurous. Try it!

Formula 3

When to Do It: This formula is excellent to address some of the common side effects of chemo relating to digestion (nausea, constipation, diarrhea, roller-coaster stomach).

How to Do It: Dissolve 2 pounds of baking soda in a tub of water as hot as can be tolerated. Stay in the bath until the water has cooled, at least 45 minutes. Do not shower for at least eight hours following the bath.

Additional: Mix ½ teaspoon of baking soda in a glass of warm water and sip this during the bath.

Formula 4

When to Do It: This formula is a general detoxifier, particularly useful to help build immunity. It is a perfect bath if you are feeling mental or emotional stress, fatigue, or for symptoms associated with the start of a cold or flu.

How to Do It: Add 2 cups of apple cider vinegar (pure, not the "flavored" variety) to a tub of water as hot as can be tolerated. Stay in the bath until the water has cooled, at least 45 minutes. Do not shower for at least eight hours following the bath.

Additional: Mix 1 tablespoon of apple cider vinegar into a glass of warm water and sip this during the bath.

Some Points to Keep in Mind

• Therapeutic bathing is most effective in the evening an hour or two before going to bed, because the body will continue to detoxify naturally during sleep.

• Use only one bathing formula per evening.

• Do not mix ingredients from different formulas; each bath is recommended only for the specific indications described.

• If redness, dryness, or roughness of the skin develops, it is an indication that the body is working to remove toxins. These aspects of cleansing are not uncommon. To minimize discomfort, rub a little olive or almond oil or a non-petroleum-based baby lotion on the skin after bathing.

Caution: If these baths are in any way too rigorous or unpleasant, please use common sense and cut back application or discontinue.

The best attitude to take toward therapeutic bathing is that it is something quite special given to us by nature to help us get back to or remain in good health. Hot springs all over the country have been sources of physical and spiritual renewal for successive generations of Native Americans and, after them, wave after wave of newcomers.

You can make your therapeutic bathing into your own personal ritual. Darken the room. Light candles. Use the time in the tub to meditate, to listen to an inspirational tape, to think, or to allow your mind to be blissfully blank. Your rituals will create a cradle of healing for yourself.

Internal: The Coffee Enema

This remarkable internal detox has been known since World War I, when, according to medical lore, nurses used left-over coffee instead of precious purified water to administer enemas to wounded soldiers.

The coffee enema is neither a colonic (colon cleanse) nor a bowel cleanse (to relieve constipation). Rather, it is a highly effective way of stimulating and detoxifying the liver and gallbladder—the body's principal organs of detoxification.

When you do the enema, coffee is transported directly to the liver by the portal vein. It's an amazing process, really. Located right above the rectum is the "S" shaped sigmoid colon. By the time the stool gets to this part of the colon, most nutrients have been absorbed back into the bloodstream. Only putrefaction products remain at this time. Now the liver and sigmoid colon work together, communicating in their own kind of circulatory-elimination system.

During a coffee enema, caffeine is sent from the end of the colon directly to the liver, where it becomes a strong detoxicant. Bile, the substance which contains much of the body's toxins, is forced to move out of the small intestine. This helps the liver to deal with even more incoming toxins from the bloodstream, organs, and tissue.

The production of an important detoxification enzyme, Glutathione-S-transferase, is also stimulated, because coffee has important alkaloids that are essential to this production. Glutathione enables toxins to be eliminated via bile into the small intestine. The result is that the detoxification process is quite rapid and effective.

The coffee enema is the king of cleanses when it comes to moving the debris accumulated in the body in the wake of a chemo treatment.

What You Need

- Enema bag with hose and catheter (the end of the hose that can be inserted into the body).

- Organic coffee, coarsely ground.

How to do it

- One quart of water—bring to a boil.

- Add 2 tablespoons organic coffee.

- Boil coffee for 5 minutes, let set until almost cool.

- Fill enema bag with the coffee.

- Lie down, insert catheter into rectum (use olive oil for lubrication if necessary), let ½ of the coffee flow in, adjusting flow with enema hose clamp.

- Retain the coffee for as long as you can, up to 12-15 minutes.

- Release, then let the rest of the coffee flow in, hold for another 12-15 minutes.

- Remember that this is not a bowel cleanse, so the coffee does not need to go farther than the very end of the colon.

- The goal of the coffee enema is to hold the coffee in for as long as you can, up to 12-15 minutes.

For even more complete directions, illustrations, and videos, please go to the website: stayhealthyduringchemo.com.

More Detox Practices

Detoxification is one of the cornerstones of good health during chemotherapy treatment. Again, I would like to emphasize the vital importance of ridding the body of the chemo cocktail mixture and the residues left after it has done its work. Here are two more detox procedures that can be done on a daily basis.

To Relieve Constipation or to Keep Toxins Moving Out

- Psyllium seed husk powder or flakes—used especially in Ayurvedic approaches to healing, this is a colon cleanse and bowel regulator. Essentially indigestible fiber, psyllium cleans the walls of the colon, collects toxins by absorption, and pushes them out of the body as a gentle laxative. You can get these at any supermarket or health food store. Follow the directions on the package.

- Magnesium citrate powder—used as a magnesium supplement, and also as a saline laxative to empty the bowels. In the body, it attracts water through osmosis and flushes out the intestines. Start with 1 level teaspoon in 8 oz. of water before bedtime and increase to a heaping teaspoon, or a bit more. The cleansing action takes place during sleep for a gentle movement in the morning. Magnesium is also responsible for over three-hundred biochemical responses in the body. It keeps everything running better.

- Hydration detox—during chemo, I advise drinking large quantities of purified water, green tea, and yerba mate to stimulate the lymphatic system, kidneys, bladder, and urinary track. The whole purpose here, remember, is to quickly rid the body of the cell-destroying chemicals and the cells they destroy.

Step 3: Eat the Best Foods to Create a Healing Chemistry in Your Body

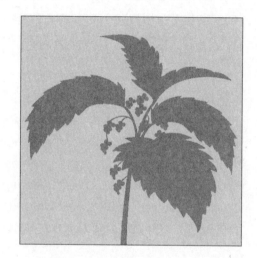

It has been my philosophy of life that difficulties vanish when faced boldly.

Isaac Asimov

At the heart of the program is the selection of the proper foods to eat during chemotherapy. There is so much misinformation out there about what foods will promote healing and which will not. Even prestigious clinics and famous cancer institutes often encourage cancer patients to eat the kind of "unrestricted diet" I described earlier.

I did a huge amount of research on the chemistry of foods for this section and found "the usual suspects" that stand in the way of healing—sugar, mostly, and foods that turn to sugar or act like sugar once they are ingested—and a few surprises, such as the tremendous healing qualities of simple green tea, ginger, cayenne pepper, and other natural herbs and spices.

These dietary recommendations are grounded on the latest nutritional studies and the cutting-edge research of medical scientists who are working to heal both cancer and the effects of chemo with what we eat.

Of all the guidelines put forth to help cancer patients undergoing chemotherapy, probably none are as full of confusion, contradiction, misunderstanding, and controversy as what to eat (food) and what to take (supplements).

In this step, I will outline what I believe is the most practical, sensible, and nutritionally and medically sound plan for the chemo diet. Virtually all the experts in the chemistry of foods, dismissing the fringe-elements on both extremes, agree on what is set out here. The main thrust of these recommendations is about changing the chemical environment within the body from a cancer-encouraging setting to a non-cancer-encouraging one.

First, here are the foods that should be avoided. To stay healthy and lessen the side effects of chemotherapy, stay away from the food list in the following pages.

Foods to Avoid

- Alcohol

- All processed foods

- Anything with artificial color or flavor added

- Deli meats and cheeses

- Caffeine

- Dairy

- Microwaved food and beverages

- Most animal protein

- Pastries, cookies, pastas, wheat

- Some oils: canola, corn, soy, palm, peanut, vegetable

- Soy beans and soy products

- Sweet fruits

- Sugar, artificial sweeteners

Alcohol

The liver processes all of the toxins in our body, including the chemicals involved in chemotherapy. By burdening liver function, alcohol can interfere with the liver's ability to effectively metabolize those toxins.

Cara Anselmo, clinical dietitian at Memorial Sloan-Kettering Cancer Center, says it's important to avoid alcohol during chemotherapy because alcohol can cause undue stress on the liver and make it harder for the liver to process chemo drugs. Alcohol can also worsen nausea or other gastrointestinal side effects.

All processed foods / Anything with artificial color or flavor added / Deli meats and cheeses

Processed foods have been altered from their natural state, usually for convenience. The methods used include canning, freezing, refrigeration, dehydration, and aseptic (sterilization) processing.

Ingredients found in processed foods contain colorants, emulsifiers, preservatives, artificial sweeteners, stabilizers, texturizers, and even bleach products, not to mention a high content of salt, sugar, and fat—all of which are counterproductive to staying healthy during chemo treatment.

According to the World Health Organization, the amounts of processed foods that are consumed are responsible for the increasing levels of obesity, heart disease, and cancer. While undergoing chemotherapy, it is vital to stay far away from the deli counter at supermarkets, avoiding bacon, sausages, ham, and lunch meats, including the self-proclaimed "healthy" varieties.

Caffeine

Caffeine dehydrates, which is just what should not happen during chemo. Dehydration contributes to the irritation of the digestive system and worsens chemo side effects, such as diarrhea and fatigue. It restricts red blood cells and depletes oxygen, and it is highly acidic.

Here I am speaking mostly about the caffeine in coffee and some soft drinks, which creates a fertile environment for cancer to thrive. Green tea and other teas contain come some caffeine, but the health-promoting qualities in green tea, especially, far out-weigh any potential downsides. (There are approximately 35-45 mg. of caffeine in a cup of green tea, compared to over 100 mg. in a similar amount of coffee.) Green tea is also high in the amino acid L-theanine, which produces both a calming effect and helps in concentration. Studies have found an association between con-suming green tea and a reduced risk for several cancers, including, skin, breast, lung, colon, and bladder.

Dairy products

"The increase in cancer, heart disease, diabetes, obesity, and asthma that has occurred in the Western world over the past cen-tury directly correlates with the increase in dairy consumption," writes Dr. Adam Meade.

Dr. T. Colin Campbell, author of *The China Study,* the most com-prehensive study of human nutrition ever conducted, says: "What protein consistently and strongly promoted cancer? Casein, which makes up 87% of cow's milk protein, promoted all stages of the cancer process. What type of protein did not promote cancer, even at high levels of intake? The safe proteins were from plants...."

Dairy products are milk (including skim, low-fat, and powdered milk), cheese, cottage cheese, cream cheese, butter, ghee, ricotta, yogurt, ice cream, gelato, and condensed or evaporated milk. If you have a question about what actually comprises "dairy," check the Internet for more complete lists.

On the subject of butter, which I consider "dairy" even though it may be technically classified as a fat: best to keep it out of the che-

motherapy diet. Butter substitutes are processed vegetable oil, usually, and therefore are nutritionally unsupportive and to be avoided.

Microwaved food and beverages

The latest research has begun to tip on the side of warning
against microwaved food and beverages. A Spanish study published in the *Journal of the Science of Food and Agriculture* noted that
87% of the nutrient value of three cancer-protecting antioxidants
(flavonoids, sinapics and caffeoyl-quinic derivatives) were lost in
microwaving.

Other studies show that the microwaving of human breast milk
destroys lysozyme, which fights bacterial infections; that microwaving destroys vitamin B-12; and that microwaving converts some
trans-amino acids into synthetic substances similar to unhealthy
trans-fatty acids. A Russian research team reported that people
who ate microwaved food had a statistically higher incidence of
stomach and intestinal cancers, digestive disorders, and lymphatic
malfunctions, causing degeneration of the immune system.

Certainly more scientific investigations need to be done on how
microwaving changes the molecular structure of foods—and what
the implications might be for human health. Meanwhile, I advise
cancer patients on chemo to avoid using the microwave oven.

Most animal protein

An up-to-the-minute report in *The New York Times* cites new research in the *Archives of Internal Medicine* implicating red meat in

the cancer scenario: "Eating red meat is associated with a sharply increased risk of death from cancer and heart disease . . . and the more of it you eat, the greater the risk."

What is stunning about the findings is that they included the remarkable conclusion that "each daily increase of three ounces of red meat was associated with a 12% greater risk of dying over all, including a 16% greater risk of cardiovascular death and a 10% greater risk of cancer death."

If the meat is processed—such as with bacon, sausages, and deli meats—the risks are even greater: "20% overall, 21% for cardiovascular disease and 16% for cancer."

To counter that report, Dr. Joseph Mercola says that the research was flawed and misrepresented. On his informative website (mercola.com), he notes,

"Trials that have compared meat-heavy diets against meat-restricted ones have consistently negated the hypothesis that meat causes disease and premature death. On the contrary, such trials have by and large found that meat-rich diets produce greater health results, such as greater weight loss, less heart disease and reduced diabetes risk."

But he is talking, remember, about how eating red meat affects healthy bodies. Most of the new research on meat with regard to cancer patients confirms what nutritional scientists have been saying for years, most convincingly in *The China Study*. For a chemo patient, eating red meat could be a risk that is just not worth taking.

Pastries, cookies, pastas, wheat

I am lumping baked goods in with wheat because virtually all familiar pastries and cookies start with wheat as the first ingredient. The second ingredient is, of course, sugar, another health hazard, which I will discuss below.

Wheat contains the complex carbohydrate amylopectin A, a starch which is very quickly digested by the body. When it enters the bloodstream, it immediately turns to sugar—at a rate more rapid than sugar itself.

So when we eat wheat, our bodies respond as if we were eating sugar. As a result, wheat's blood sugar implication contributes heavily to many common health problems: obesity, diabetes, cardiovascular disease, hypo- and hyperglycemia, and many other ailments.

Furthermore, wheat contains the protein gluten, which can damage the lining of the small intestine. When that happens, nutrients are absorbed poorly and unwanted proteins can come into the body—resulting in an overtaxing of the immune system.

The New England Journal of Medicine lists fifty-five diseases that can be caused by eating gluten, including osteoporosis, irritable bowel disease, inflammatory bowel disease, anemia, cancer, fatigue, canker sores, rheumatoid arthritis, lupus, multiple sclerosis, and almost all other autoimmune diseases. Gluten is also linked to many psychiatric and neurological diseases, including anxiety, depression, and schizophrenia.

Please note that regular pasta products are made of wheat, so they should be avoided. Rice pastas (noodles) are fine, of course.

Some oils

The only acceptable oils for the chemotherapy diet are extra virgin olive oil, coconut oil, avocado oil, and walnut oil. Of these, only olive oil and coconut oil can be heated in the cooking and food preparation process; avocado and walnut oil should be used in their natural, unheated state.

Avoid canola oil, palm oil, vegetable oil, corn oil, peanut oil, and soy oil. Canola oil (rapeseed oil) was produced in the 19th century as a lubricant for steam engines; it is one of the first ingredients in commercial bug sprays. Palm oil has been shown to clog arteries. Peanut oil—along with peanuts themselves—should be avoided because peanuts contain many fungi that can interfere with immune system function.

Corn, soy, and vegetable oils are the lowest grade oils; they contain no nutritional benefits whatever. Conventional vegetable oil is similar to junk food because it is processed—and, in fact, it is widely used in the preparation of junk food. During the production stage, most of the few nutrients it had to begin with are extracted, leaving only the oil. This means that when people consume vegetable oil, they are consuming nothing but useless fat.

One of the additional hidden dangers of vegetable oils is that many of them are genetically modified. Corn, soybean, canola, and cottonseed oils are the top genetically modified vegetable oils in the United States. Obviously, these have no place in a healthy diet for a cancer patient.

Soy beans and soy products

Dr. Kaayla Daniel, author of the groundbreaking book *The Whole Soy Story: The Dark Side of America's Favorite Health Food*, points to thousands of studies implicating soy in digestive problems, immune-system breakdown, thyroid dysfunction, cognitive decline, reproductive disorders—even heart disease and cancer, particularly breast cancer.

Dr. Joseph Mercola, citing Dr. Daniel, says that "Ninety-one percent of soy grown in the US is genetically modified (GMO). The genetic modification is done to impart resistance to the toxic herbicide Roundup. While this is meant to increase farming efficiency and provide you with less expensive soy, the downside is that your soy is loaded with this toxic pesticide." And Dr. Daniel adds that "going 'organic' does not make soy healthy; it's just that GMO is worse."

Soy beans and soy products (tofu, soy powder in "health drinks," soy milk, soy oil) are difficult to avoid, by the way, since soy is now an ingredient in so many processed foods, such as chocolate, cookies, salad dressings, soups, sauces, margarine, and vegetarian meat substitutes. But it is essential that a cancer patient on chemotherapy stay away from soy, mainly because it compromises the immune system—exactly what must not happen during cancer treatment. I advise you to get in the habit of reading ingredient lists and to be particularly on the lookout for hidden soy in foods.

Fermented soy products such as natto, tempeh, and soy sauce are acceptable soy choices, but should be eaten in moderation because of their high acid content.

Sweet Fruits

Avoid all sweet fruits, such as mangos, nectarines, oranges, peaches, yellow apples, tangerines, grapes, honeydew, figs, plums, and dates. Their high glycemic content makes them not a good choice in a diet for anyone undergoing chemotherapy. Sweet fruit (fresh or dried) turns into instant energy for all cells, including cancer cells. It is best to keep all sugar-related foods out of the diet. One quick note: raisins, although a dried fruit, are considered a "lesser evil," and may be used sparingly.

A quick note here: nutritional scientists are investigating the enzyme bromelain, which is extracted from pineapple stems. Bromelain is selectively cytotoxic—that is, it will kill cancer cells, but not healthy cells—and was shown to be superior to the chemotherapy drug 5-fluorauracil in treating cancer in animal tests.

Sugar, artificial sweeteners

Volumes have been written about the health dangers of eating sugar. I will only make a couple of points here, relating them specifically to cancer treatment. By the way, I include all artificial sweeteners here, because they act exactly like sugar in the body.

When we eat sugar, the pancreas is stimulated to secrete insulin in order to drop blood-sugar levels. The result is a rapid fluctuation of blood-sugar levels, which places a great deal of stress on the body. Sugar raises the insulin level in the body, which inhibits the release of growth hormones—which in turn depresses the immune system. For someone coping with cancer and chemotherapy, depressing the immune system must be avoided at all costs.

The sugar-insulin-immune system connection is the primary reason to remove sugar (including hidden sugars in processed foods) entirely from the diet. But there is more. Sugar can:

- contribute to anxiety, depression, and concentration difficulties

- upset the body's mineral balance

- cause kidney damage

- contribute to a weakened defense against bacterial infection

- increase the amount of fat in the liver, the body's main organ for detoxing dead cancer cells and chemo chemicals

- cause liver cells to divide, increasing the size of the liver.

Cancer cells are nourished primarily on sugar. To detect where a tumor may be present in the body, we use PET scans that simply measure where radioactive sugar accumulates.

I could go on and on with the list. The bottom line of my advice goes back to the nutritional wisdom we have been living with for a hundred years, sometimes forgotten in modern times: sugar feeds cancer.

A diet for someone on chemotherapy should include the food types in the proportions shown in the chart.

Daily Menu Planner

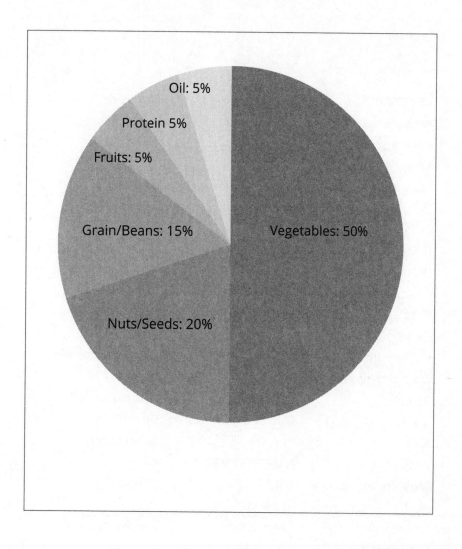

Foods to Enjoy

 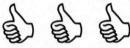

VEGETABLES
Artichokes
Asparagus
Arugula
Avocados
Bell pepper, red & yellow
Bok choy
Broccoli
Brussels sprouts
Cabbage
Cauliflower
Collard greens
Dark leafy greens
Fennel
Garlic
Kale
Leeks
Mushrooms, shii-take
Onions
Sea vegetables
Spinach
Sprouts
Sweet potatoes
Swiss chard

FRUITS
Apples, green
Blackberries
Blueberries
Boysenberries
Lemon/limes
Pomegranates
Raspberries

MILKS
Almond Milk (unsweetened)
Oat Milk

NUTS, SEEDS & OILS
Almonds
Cashews
Chia seeds
Coconut oil, organic
Extra virgin olive oil
Flaxseeds
Pumpkin seeds
Walnuts

GRAINS
Brown rice
Quinoa

SPICES & HERBS
Basil
Cayenne pepper
Chili peppers
Cilantro/coriander seeds
Cinnamon, ground
Cumin seeds
Fennel seeds
Ginger
Oregano
Parsley
Peppermint
Rosemary
Spirulina

VEGETABLES

Bell pepper, green
Corn
Cucumbers
Green beans
Mustard/turnip greens
Rhubarb
Squash
Tomatoes

SEAFOOD

Cod
Sardines
Scallops
Shrimp

FRUITS

Apricots
Cherries
Cranberries
Grapefruit
Strawberries

BEANS & LEGUMES

Black beans
Garbanzo beans (chickpeas)
Lentils

NUTS, SEEDS & OILS

Sesame seeds

GRAINS

Buckwheat
Oats
Rye

SPICES & HERBS

Black pepper
Garlic
Mustard seeds
Sage
Thyme

SEAFOOD

Halibut
Salmon
Tuna

FRUITS

Apples, red
Bananas, green
Raisins
Watermelon

EGGS & MILK

Eggs
Milk, goat
Yogurt, goat

BEANS & LEGUMES

Kidney beans
Lima beans
Navy beans
Pinto beans

POULTRY & LEAN MEATS

Lamb (if anemic)

GRAIN

Barley

NATURAL SWEETENERS

Blackstrap molasses

Neutral or Less Beneficial

VEGETABLES
Beets
Carrots
Celery
Edamame
Iceberg lettuce
Okra

Olives
Peas

POULTRY & LEAN MEATS
Chicken
Turkey

NATURAL SWEETENERS
Agave nectar
Stevia

NOTE: You will see right away that the diet I consider most beneficial for a cancer patient going through chemotherapy is almost entirely plant-based. I have drawn these recommendations from recent nutritional studies, foremost among them the revolutionary *The China Study* by T. Colin Campbell. When it came out, *The New York Times* called it "Grand Prix of epidemiology" because of the length and breadth of its scope: it examined more than 350 variables of health and nutrition with surveys from 6,500 adults in more than 2,500 counties across China and Taiwan. The study presents impressive evidence that a low-protein, low-glycemic, plant-based diet is best to prevent and recover from cancer.

The China Study is controversial, nonetheless, with its critics calling some of the research into question, even flawed by an enthusiasm to present plant-based eating in the best light. They cite the work of pioneering integrative oncologists who are experimenting with "metabolic typing"—recommending a diet that matches the metabolism of the individual patient, sometimes including red meat. These investigations are also compelling.

Still, Campbell's findings in his twenty-year study seem sensible to me. I personally follow these guidelines as much as possible and recommend them to my clients as a healthy way of eating.

Additional Things to Consider

- Organic, organic, organic: whenever possible, purchase organic varieties of the recommended foods.

- As much as possible, eat only "whole foods"—foods with only one ingredient.

- The "well-balanced diet" is a myth perpetrated by people who are ignorant about the chemistry of foods; disregard pie-charts and pyramids showing that you need red meat, wheat, and dairy products to stay healthy.

- Cooking vegetables: steam, don't boil or fry. Boiling water leaches nutrients from vegetables, and heat destroys nutrients in oil.

- Enjoy your food, eat slowly for the sake of good digestion and assimilation, feel the life-giving nutrients you are taking into your body.

- Grow your own: sprouts (one of the most nutritious foods you can eat) and wheat grass (also very nutritious) are easy to grow and harvest. Visit the website for video demonstrations: stayhealthyduringchemo.com.

Step 4: Supplement Your Diet Correctly to Support the Healing Momentum

Every crucial experience can be regarded as a setback - or the start of a new kind of development.

Mary Roberts Kinehart

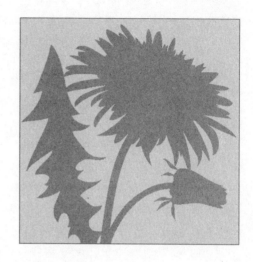

If "what shall I eat?" is the first big area of concern to chemo patients, surely the next has to be "what shall I take?" in terms of supplements in the form of vitamins, minerals and herbs. Again, I found this to be a subject with an enormous amount of confusion and controversy attached to it.

Citing studies that look and sound reputable, some oncologists say that certain vitamins, minerals, and herbal compounds will lessen the effects of chemotherapy or interfere with its work. Other oncologists, referring to research just as well-grounded in good science over many years, tell us that taking food supplements makes no difference whatever during chemotherapy. The new "integrative oncologists"—cancer doctors who include holistic approaches along with traditional treatments—say that supplements enhance the effectiveness of chemotherapy and help the body to heal faster from both cancer and the immune-suppression work of chemo, and extend survival rates.

In this book, I'm suggesting a generous round of supplementation. The kind of supplements and the recommended dosage, you'll see, are "therapeutic" in nature, designed to help push toxins out of the body and repair and fortify the immune system.

Should or should we not supplement a chemo patient's diet with vitamins, minerals, and herbs, especially those with high antioxidant values? The invariable direction from most conventional oncologists is to refrain from supplements during chemotherapy treatment. Some, believing supplements are basically ineffective and therefore harmless, will allow them during treatment—but not on the day chemo is administered.

The argument, and the controversy, is that supplements may produce chemical changes in the body that will interfere in some way with the work of the chemotherapy drugs. At the heart of the debate is whether antioxidants feed the growth of normal cells or cancer cells, or both at the same time. Antioxidants, you will remember, are nutrients in foods which prevent or slow the oxidative damage to our body. These nutrients can be extracted from foods and are available in concentrated form as supplements.

Proponents of the no-supplement idea believe that taking them may impede the efforts of chemotherapy to destroy cancer cells. But advocates of supplements point out that antioxidants are already present in the food that cancer patients are eating. Moreover, they call attention to a mounting stack of new research showing that supplements, far from interfering with chemo, increase survival rates, help to reduce tumors, and enhance immunity during treatment.

Perhaps the most well-known recent research is that of Keith Block, MD, Medical Director of the Block Center for Integrative Cancer Treatment in Evanston, IL. The outcome of his research was published in 2008 in the *International Journal of Cancer.*

Dr. Block and his team undertook two systematic reviews of the medical literature and concluded that there is no evidence to support the theory that antioxidant supplements interfere with the therapeutic effects of chemotherapy agents. Furthermore, they found that antioxidants improve treatment outcomes, expand survival times, and increase tumor responses. Thus, antioxidants and chemotherapy are safely recommended for metastatic and palliative care patients. (Much of this information is contained in the excellent book that Dr. Block authored with Dr. Andrew Weil in 2007, *Life Over Cancer: The Block Center Program for Integrative Cancer Treatment.*)

Michael Lam, M.D., M.P.H., A.B.A.A.M., concurs, telling us, "Fortunately, a large body of evidence is available to show a positive effect of high dose repeated use of antioxidants in the period before, during and after conventional cancer therapy."

Dr. Andrew Weil is more cautious, but in general supports supplementation during chemotherapy, suggesting that a patient "[not] take antioxidant supplements on the day before, the day of, and the day after chemotherapy; otherwise, it is okay to take supplements."

Abram Hoffer, M.D., Ph.D., a colleague of Dr. Linus Pauling, the Nobel Laureate who promoted megavitamin therapy for health and longevity, enthusiastically supported the use of supplements during cancer treatment. In a well-known essay, he cites the work of Dr. Kedar N. Prasad, whose review of seventy-one scientific papers, "found no evidence that antioxidants...interfere with the therapeutic effect of chemotherapy and, on the contrary, suggest the hypothesis that it would increase the efficacy."

Dr. Hoffer goes on to mention the earlier research of Charles B. Simone, M.MS., M.D., who came to the same conclusion. He quotes Dr. Simone, "In a recent study of 50 patients with early-stage breast cancer I evaluated the treatment side effects of radiation alone, or radiation combined with chemotherapy, while the patients took therapeutic doses of nutrients. Patients were asked to evaluate their own response to the treatment in terms of its impact on their quality of life. The results of the study were impressive: more than 90% of both groups noted improvement in their physical symptoms, cognitive ability, performance, sexual function, general well-being and life satisfaction. Not one subject in either group reported a worsening of symptoms."

I support the side that advances the new science, all of which is indicating that application of supplements in chemotherapy treatment is beneficial. If you would like to go deeper into the question of supplements, I encourage you to check out the articles about this important topic that I've collected on our website.

Visit the website: stayhealthyduringchemo.com

Supplement Summary

For a person already enjoying good health and eating a great diet of a variety of whole foods, and living a low-stress lifestyle, a simple comprehensive multivitamin and mineral may be enough to maintain well-being. But a cancer patient undergoing chemotherapy and other cancer treatments needs much more to help deal with both the original malady and the conventional chemical remedies used to address it.

In this section, I recommend therapeutic doses of supplements that specifically address the healing process during chemo. It may seem like a lot, but each is valuable to stay healthy while in treatment—and beyond.

Here they are, from A to Z. My recommended dosage per day is [in brackets]. Where more than one per day is indicated, try to take the additional capsules or tablets at different times throughout the day. These are all recommended dosages for adults; for children, quantities should be halved, or check with the main health care provider. Remember that unless specified, supplements always get into the body faster and better when taken with food.

- Alpha Lipoic Acid—200 mg [3]

- Biotin—5000 mcg [2]

- CoQ10—100 mg [2]

- Multi-Vitamin and Mineral—[1]

- Niacin (Vitamin B3)—1000 mg, flush-free [2]

- Omega 3/Fish Oil—1000 mg [1]

- Panax Ginseng—500 mg [3]

- Pancreatin 8x [1] + 4x [4]

- Selenium—200 mcg [1]

- Spirulina—500 mg [4]

- Vitamin B Complex—50 mg [2]

- Vitamin C—1000 mg [3] or more, depending on bowel tolerance

- Vitamin D3—5000 IU [1]

- Vitamin E—400 IU [2]

- Zinc—50 mg [2]

On the website, I've listed all these supplements and, to make it easy for you to get them, you'll find information about manufacturers and distributors of what I consider the highest quality supplements. Visit: stayhealthyduringchemo.com

Annotated Supplement List

Here are more details on the supplements I am recommending, with special reference to why they should be part of a program of healing for chemotherapy patients.

Alpha Lipoic Acid—Alpha lipoic acid is an antioxidant that is made by the body and is found in every cell. Other antioxidants work only in water (such as vitamin C) or fatty tissues (such as vitamin E), but alpha lipoic acid is both fat- and water-soluble, which means it can work throughout the body. Antioxidants are used up as they attack free radicals, but research is showing that alpha lipoic acid may help regenerate these other antioxidants and make them active again.

Biotin—Biotin, a super metabolizer, processes carbohydrates, protein, and fat quickly. Especially good for sluggish systems brought on by some of the side effects of chemo, such as fatigue and constipation.

CoQ10—A highly effective antioxidant that boosts the immune system and protects heart function.

Multi-Vitamin and Mineral—A comprehensive multi-vitamin and mineral as a general supplemental support. This is especially important given the ups and downs of appetite during chemo.

Niacin (Vitamin B3)—Flush-free niacin is a strong antioxidant and detoxifier, involved in over 50 metabolic processes that turn carbohydrates into energy.

Omega 3/Fish Oil—Omega 3 is an essential fatty acid that is a natural anti-inflammatory and helps with nervous system function. DHA, an omega 3 fatty acid found in fish oils, has been shown to reduce the size of tumors and enhance the positive effects of the chemotherapy drug cisplatin, while limiting its harmful side effects.

Panax Ginseng—A highly effective stimulant especially for mental activity and a general tonic. Specifically, ginseng can help to lessen the effects of "chemo brain," improving thinking and memory functions.
Follow safety precautions on the package and use responsibly, especially if you have a history of endocrine disorders or high blood pressure.

Pancreatin—A group of enzymes that break down protein thus helping to irradicate cancer. This is described more fully on the next page.

Selenium—Selenium works with the body's natural antioxidant, glutathione. It also works in tandem with Vitamin E to protect the outer walls of cells.

Spirulina—Spirulina is a blue-green algae that grows in warm, watery and highly alkaline environments. It comes in powdered form, also in capsules and tablets. Spirulina is essentially chlorophyll, the green pigment in plants, a potent detoxifier and immune system booster.

Vitamin B Complex—The B vitamins (except B1, thiamine, which can speed cell division) are important especially to help with stress and to keep energy up.

Vitamin C—Vitamin C is water-soluble, which means that it is not stored in the body, and passes through rather quickly. It comes as powder, crystals, or capsules. A great antioxidant.

Vitamin D3—This can slow the growth of cancer cells and boosts immunity.

Vitamin E—Studies have shown that this vital antioxidant can thwart the growth of cancer cells, while at the same time boosting immunity.

Zinc—Zinc, an antioxidant mineral, helps build and repair cells and tissues, and enhances immunity (which is why we take zinc at the first sign of a cold).

A Special Case: Enzyme Therapy

More about pancreatin and proteolytic enzymes in general:

Enzymes are proteins that help us digest our food and act as catalysts for almost every cellular activity in our bodies. Proteolytic enzymes are produced by the pancreas, which sends digestive enzymes to the small intestines.

Proteolytic enzymes, taken on an empty stomach, are able to break down the walls of cancer cells and allow the immune system to get rid of them easily. These enzymes, which also digest complete proteins, remove the protein coating on cancer cell walls, leaving the cancer cells defenseless against the immune system.

There is a fascinating history to proteolytic enzyme therapy and the healing of cancer. It began in 1911 with the work of John Beard, a Scottish embryologist, who made a connection between enzymes and cancer cells, and successfully experimented on eliminating cancer in animals and humans with injections of pancreatic juices.

Forty years later the idea was taken up again by William Donald Kelley, who healed his own pancreatic cancer, then proceeded to cure patients with other forms of cancer. From Kelley, we move in a direct line to Dr. Nicholas Gonzalez, who is currently practicing enzyme therapy on cancer patients in clinical trials using his own specially prepared proteolytic enzymes and metabolic therapy.

To see several articles on this subject, with links to all the most recent studies, check our website: stayhealthyduringchemo.com.

Always tell your health care provider what you are taking to be sure there are no undesirable side effects. Chemotherapy patients should check with their doctors about taking angelica, arnica, bogbean, boldo, celery supplements, clove oil, danshen, feverfew, ginkgo, onion supplements, papain, and willow bark as these might impact some treatments.

My Own Herbal Formula

This is a herbal formula I created from the research I did on the specific topic of immune support during cancer treatment. This is a powerful blend that can speed up the healing process by combining cleansing with increased stamina and immune building.

Cell Support Formula

All of these ingredients are to be combined and used in powder form. I am using "parts" to denote a general measuring method. If you are using a tablespoon, "one part" would be one tablespoon; if a scoop, then "one part" is one scoop, and so on. Best is to mix them together thoroughly in a large mixing bowl.

Dosage: take 2 tablespoons 3 times per day mixed in a glass of water, spaced throughout the day. Avoid taking close to bedtime.

Cell Support Formula

Asparagus (1 part)	Astragalus (2 parts)
Bio flavonoids (2 parts)	Cayenne (1/8 part)
Goldenseal (1/4 part)	Magnesium (1-1/4 parts)
Maitake mushroom (2 parts)	Reishi mushrooms (2 parts)
Schizandra berry (1 part)	Spinach (1 part)

Annotated Cell Support List

The descriptions of these herbal powders come from several sources in books and on the Internet. Find direct links to these on our website: stayhealthyduringchemo.com.

Asparagus—Asparagus contains the highest amount of the highly valued antioxidant glutathione. Glutathione protects the body against certain types of cancer, boosts the immune system, and defends against particular viruses. It also helps to fight fatigue, exhaustion, and joint pain.

Astragalus—This herb helps treat cancer through enhancing the immune system. Astragalus contains polysaccharides, such as selenium, which are active and effective elements that increase T-cells. (T-cells, short for Thymus cells, are white blood cells that are important in maintaining the body's immune system, and are essential in fighting harmful invading substances.) Astragalus also helps protect cells of cancer patients from more harm caused by the disease, especially from toxics and metals they may be subjected to during treatment.

Dr. Oz recommends astragalus as part of his anti-aging program because of the herb's adaptogen (a substance that helps the body regenerate after being fatigued or stressed) properties.

Bio flavonoids—These chemicals provide a huge dose of antioxidant help to our internal systems. Flavonoids also have a low toxicity level compared to other active plant compounds. They have been called "nature's biological response modifiers" because they can help us react appropriately to viruses, carcinogens, and allergens by giving a powerful boost to the immune system. Flavonoids exhibit anti-inflammatory, anti-microbial, and anti-cancer properties because they protect against oxidative and free radical damage caused by pollution and the body's normal metabolic processes.

Cayenne—This miracle pepper is nothing short of amazing for its effects on the circulatory system, as it feeds vital elements into the cell structure of capillaries, veins, arteries, and helps adjust blood pressure to normal levels. Cayenne cleans the arteries as well, helping to rid the body of the "bad" LDL cholesterol and triglycerides.

Cayenne is also great for the stomach and the intestinal tract. It stimulates the peristaltic motion of the intestines and aids in assimilation and elimination. In clinical studies conducted in Japan, England, and the United States, capsaicin, the critical secondary metabolite compound found in cayenne pepper, has been shown to cause cancer cells to undergo "apoptosis"—cell suicide.

Goldenseal—Goldenseal's numerous uses are attributed to its antibiotic, anti-inflammatory, and astringent properties. It soothes irritated mucus membranes, aiding the eyes, ears, nose, and throat. Taken at the first signs of respiratory problems, colds, or flu, goldenseal helps prevent further symptoms from developing. It has also been used to help reduce fevers, and relieve congestion and excess mucus.

Goldenseal cleanses and promotes healthy glandular functions by increasing bile flow and digestive enzymes, and by doing so, regulates healthy liver and spleen functions. It can relieve constipation and may also be used to treat infections of the bladder and intestines as well.

Goldenseal contains calcium, iron, manganese, vitamin A, vitamin C, vitamin E, B-complex, and other nutrients and minerals. The roots and rhizomes of goldenseal contain many isoquinoline alkaloids, including hydrastine, berberine, canadine, canadaline, and l-hydrastine as well as traces of essential oil, fatty oil, and resin. It is believed that the high content of these alkaloids gives goldenseal its antibiotic, anti-infective, and immune stimulating qualities.

Magnesium—Magnesium is the second most abundant element inside human cells and the fourth most abundant positively charged ion in the human body. Within the body's cells, it serves more than 300 functions. From relaxing muscle tissue to sharpening brain function, magnesium is an essential mineral for restoring and maintaining health.

Bestselling author Daniel Reid tell us that "Magnesium is particularly important as a co-factor in maintaining functional balance in the nervous and endocrine systems, and it's an indispensable element in all of the body's natural self-cleansing and detoxification responses. Without sufficient magnesium, toxic waste and acid residues accumulate in cells and tissues, setting the stage for chronic degenerative conditions, cancer, and rapid aging symptoms."

Maitake Mushroom—This mushroom has proven itself to be an effective cancer fighter. In laboratory tests, powdered maitake increased the activity of three types of immune cells-macrophages, natural killer (NIK) cells, and T-cells by 140%, 186%, and 160%, respectively. Researchers have found that maitake, when combined with the standard chemotherapy drug mitomycin (mutamycin), inhibits the growth of breast cancer cells, even after metastasis.

Studies have shown that maitake can induce interferon production which may have an effect if you are on a strict interferon prescription. Please consult your practitioner if you are on such an interferon prescription.

Reishi Mushroom—The water-soluble polysaccharides, beta-glucans and hetero-beta-glucans, are active ingredients found in the red reishi mushroom. These polysaccharides boost the immune system, fight tumors, and lower blood pressure. Reishi also contains the ling zhi-8 protein, which is an immune system booster.

Supplementing with reishi is considered to be very safe, but patients undergoing organ transplants or using immunosuppressive drugs should be careful because any immune-modulating substance can interact adversely.

Schizandra Berry—This "power" berry comes from China—its Chinese name is wu-wei-zi, which means five taste fruit. Double blind studies suggest that schizandra has the ability to help those who suffer from hepatitis. The lignans in the berry appear to protect the liver by stimulating cells that produce much-needed antioxidants. Because of its adaptogenic properties, it has been applied next to some herbal medicines, such as ginseng, as a stimulator for the central nervous system, increased brain efficiency, improved reflexes, and an accelerated rate of endurance.

Spinach—According to Popeye, as we all know, spinach contributes to good health. And new research confirms it. One new category of health-supportive nutrients found in spinach is called "glycoglycerolipids." Glycoclycerolipids are the main fat-related molecules in the membranes of light-sensitive organs in most plants.

Recent studies in laboratory animals have shown that glyco-glycerolipids from spinach can help protect the lining of the digestive tract from damage—especially damage related to unwanted inflammation.

Certain unique anti-cancer carotenoids—called epoxyxantho-phylls—are plentiful in spinach, and they are almost as effectively absorbed as other carotenoids like beta-carotene and lutein.

A Final Word

Drug companies that produce chemotherapy chemicals put out a list of what is called absolute or relative contraindication—that is, a certain substance should not be taken at the same time a particular chemo drug is taken because of the specific chemical properties of each. Your oncologist will know about these and will tell you about them, but remember to ask.

Step 5: Exercise and Rest to Speed the Healing Process

Therefore choose life!

Bible, Deuteronomy 30:19

Body movement may seem the furthest thing from a chemo patient's mind, but a certain amount of exercise is part of the prescription for healing. Gentle movement will energize the body's ability to dispel toxins and assimilate the high-octane nutrition from food and supplements. More than 100 studies involving cancer survivors show that exercise is associated with lower cancer recurrences rates and lengthier survival rates.

I'm presenting two types of exercise in this step. One is a series of easy-to-learn and easy-to-practice yoga-type movements. The other is simple walking, a great tonic not only for the physical body, but also for the mind and emotions.

A chemo patient shouldn't need to be told how important it is to rest—many may feel that they are resting most of the time, just from feeling the fatigue that is one of the side effects of chemotherapy. But resting is a huge part of the healing process, the time when the real body-mending takes place. In this section, I recommend ways to rest deeply as a health-giving practice.

A new study conducted at two university hospitals in Denmark confirms other research into the effects of exercise on cancer patients. Exercise, both of high and low intensity, not only could be safely used during chemotherapy treatment, but was found to reduce fatigue and improve vitality, aerobic capacity, muscular strength, and physical activity—and expand emotional well-being.

In this section, I recommend two excellent forms of exercise that are easy to do and will "move things around" to help speed up the healing process.

The Tibetan Rites

So much has been written about the amazing Five Tibetan Rites—do an Internet search, and over 50,000 sites will come up. They have been known for many years—some say many centuries—and occasionally take on new popularity, as they did recently when they were demonstrated by Dr. Oz on his TV show.

I'm going to outline some information on the Rites and their health benefits here and then suggest that you go to our own website for videos demonstrating the exact way to do them.

The Tibetan Rites are five easy yoga-like positions that are done once or more every day. Together, they take only about 10-15 minutes to perform.

Briefly, according to the Tibetan lamas, the only difference between youth and old age is the spin rate of the chakras, the body's seven major energy centers. The chakras turn at high speed in a healthy, youthful body. As we get older, the chakras slow down and the body is open to illness and starts to show signs of aging. We can regain youth, vitality, and good health, by getting the chakras to spin at a higher rate, as they did when we were much younger.

The benefits of doing the Tibetan Rites are many: improved general health, more energy, better clarity of thinking and improvement in memory, less stress, a higher sense of well-being, calm, and a more positive outlook. For cancer patients, the Rites not only speed up the healing process by activating the body's energy centers, but they also provide much-needed physical activity to move things around inside, and move toxins out of, the body.

Each of the five positions is repeated 21 times—you start out with 3 or 5 (always an odd-number) and gradually work up to 21 over several days or weeks.

The illustrations on the next pages show what the positions look like.

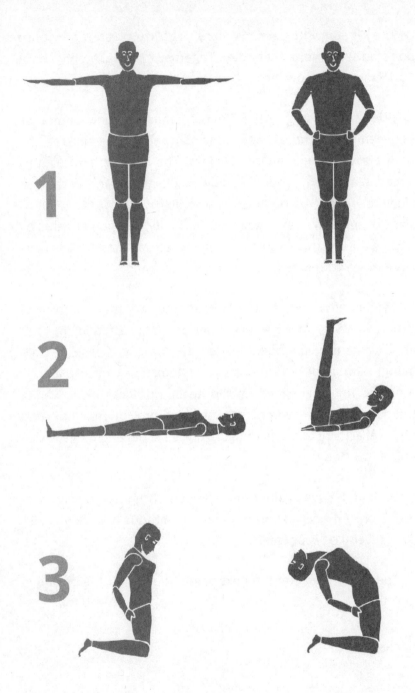

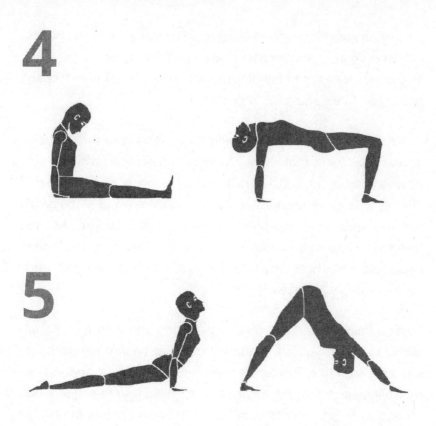

To see the Five Tibetan Rites explained further and demonstrated in videos, go to our website: stayhealthyduringchemo.com.

Walking

The second exercise I recommend is simple walking. Surely this has to be the easiest—and least expensive—exercise in the world. It is also one of the most important activities for a person in chemo treatment to embrace.

In my study of the literature of cancer healing, time and again walking comes up as a way to keep bones, muscles, and joints healthy and working right. Walking also reduces anxiety and wards off depression—two persistent bugaboos for cancer patients. It also makes it easier to handle stress, to sleep better and deeper, and to feel more energetic in general.

Finally, walking is good for self-esteem. This is so for a couple of reasons. One is that when you finish a walk, you have a sense of accomplishment, and that makes you feel better about yourself. The other is more chemical in nature. Walking—and all physical exercise—releases endorphins into the system. Endorphins are feel-good chemicals produced by the pituitary gland and the hypothalamus. That's why it feels so good to move around. And for a cancer patient, feeling good is good!

As a final point, if you take a walk every day with a friend or family member, you are giving yourself the opportunity to have more of a social life. This can be tremendously helpful in addressing the solitary and isolating nature of illness. Being with and around other people gets us outside of ourselves and more into the swing of life.

Resting

Finally, let me say something about resting. I consider resting an important "activity" when it is done with purpose and mindfulness.

Most of the time, a cancer patient undergoing chemo, radiation, and other conventional therapies will rest just because there is no energy to do anything else. There are times, though, when one has a choice to remain in a kind of semi-active state or to lie down and rest. My advice is that instead of continuing to putter around the house or push yourself into physical activities, lie down and rest.

Rest is the time when the body does the greater part of healing. While you are moving around, your body is busy expending the energy it takes to stand, bend, reach, climb, pace, and so on. Even light housekeeping, tidying up the bedroom and bathroom or wiping off the kitchen counter, takes energy that might better be used for mending while at rest.

One of the reasons I mention resting here is because I have heard from cancer patients that they sometimes feel guilty that they are not busy doing things—that they might be seen as lazy or entitled, especially when measuring themselves against their tireless caregiver, who appears to be working diligently on their behalf every minute of the day.

Nonsense. If you are going through cancer treatment, no one expects you to be full of pep and up to your usual activities. Rest is a blessing. As you drift off to sleep in the middle of the day, you may want to recall as you sink into repose that resting is your way of continuing your courageous journey of healing.

PART THREE

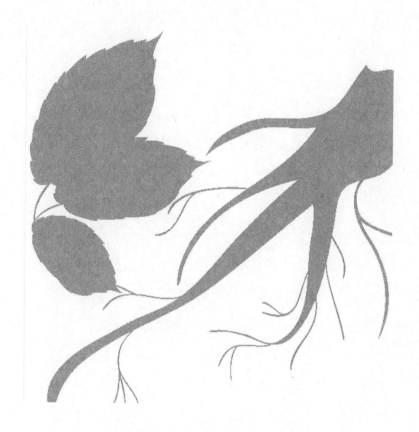

Recipes: Eating Healthy

PART THREE

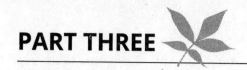

Recipes: Eating Healthy

> The longer I live, the less confidence I have in drugs and the greater is my confidence in the regulation and administration of diet and regimen.
>
> *John Redman Coxe, 1800*

> We are indeed much more than what we eat, but what we eat can nevertheless help us to be much more than what we are.
>
> *Adelle Davis (1904-1974)*

BASICS

Foods to Prepare Ahead of Time and Keep on Hand

Cooked Beans—can keep in the refrigerator for up to a week. The easiest way to cook dried beans is to clean and wash them thoroughly, put in a slow-cooker, add 2-1/2 cups of water for each cup of beans. Cook overnight on the lowest setting.

Alternative: clean and wash, soak in water overnight. In the morning, discard the soaking water (it contains much of the "gas" associated with beans). Boil over moderate heat on

STAY HEALTHY DURING CHEMO

stove top until tender—time will depend on the type of bean. Skim off foam during cooking. Add water from time to time to compensate for evaporation.

Brown Rice—make a 3-day supply and use not only for rice dishes, but also in soups or to sprinkle on salads.

Follow cooking directions on the package. If buying in bulk, allow about 2-1/2 cups of water for each cup of rice. Bring water to a boil, add rice, bring to boil again, cover and simmer for about 30 minutes.

Vegetable Broth—add to soups or use as a sipping consommé by itself. Simmer together in a very large soup pot: carrots, celery, onions, garlic, and potatoes. After about an hour, turn off heat and let set for another hour. Drain off the liquid for use, dispose of the vegetables.

Sprouts—use practically any bean or seed. Best seeds: alfalfa, clover. Best beans: mung, lentil, garbanzo. Best nuts: almonds, filberts (hazelnuts). Best grains: wheat berries, rye.

Cover in water and soak overnight. The next day, drain and place beans or seeds in a large glass jar, covered with cheesecloth fastened with a rubber band. Over the next few days, cover with water for a few minutes, then drain off. Sprouts will begin to appear in 2-3 days. Keep irrigating and draining. Sprouts may be used during the sprouting process. When they have reached maturity, refrigerate to retard the growing process.

Almond Milk and Oat Milk—to make milk of almonds or oats, soak a cup of the nuts or the oats in 2-3 cups of water overnight. In the morning, blend the contents of the bowl and strain. What are left are the milk and the pulp. Add 1/4 teaspoon of vanilla (optional) to the milk. Save the pulp and add to smoothies, cookies, and other dishes. Avoid most store-bought almond milk varieties (quickly becoming a nutritional fad), which can be filled with sugar and artificial flavors.

Oats and Gluten The subject of whether oats can be included in a gluten-free diet has been a topic of debate among health care providers. Though registered dietitian Leslie Beck states that oat flour is gluten-free, oats do contain a protein called avenin that may be toxic to some people who cannot tolerate gluten. According to an article published in the September 2006 issue of *Practical Gastroenterology,* adverse reactions to oats may be caused by cross-contamination of oat products with gluten-rich grains such as wheat or barley.

Oat Flour Oat flour is made by grinding oat groats, the whole, hulled grains of the oat plant, into a fine powder. It is often mixed with flours that contain gluten to enhance its ability to rise when baked. By itself, you must use oat flour carefully. Overdoing the mixing can deplete oxygen and carbon dioxide from the mixture, resulting in a product that fails to stick together, or that is heavy due to failure to rise, according to the cooking site, "Ellen's Kitchen."

NOTE: Oven temperatures in all the recipes that follow are in degrees Fahrenheit.

Notes

BREAKFAST

Granola

8 c. rolled oats

1 c. unsweetened flaked coconut

1/2 c. unsalted sunflower seeds

1/2 c. sesame seeds

1 c. almonds, chopped

1/2 c. coconut oil

1/2 tsp. sea salt

1 tsp. vanilla extract

Stevia, pinch

Preheat the oven to 325 degrees.

In a large bowl, stir together the oats, coconut, sunflower seeds, and almonds. In a separate bowl, mix together the oil, salt, stevia, and vanilla. Pour the liquid ingredients into the dry ingredients, and stir until evenly coated. Spread in a thin layer on a large baking sheet.

Bake for about 30-40 minutes in the preheated oven. Stir every 5-10 minutes, until lightly toasted and fragrant. When cooked, granola will be more crispy and crunchy.

Serve with cold or heated almond milk or oat milk.

Servings: 10-15

Green Apple Ginger Oatmeal

1 Granny Smith apple, cored and chopped
1 c. rolled oats (not instant)
2 c. purified water
1/2 tsp. ginger powder
1/2 tsp. cinnamon powder
Pinch of sea salt

In a medium saucepan, add all ingredients and cook over a medium heat. Stir occasionally. Add almond milk or water if consistency is too thick.

Serving: 1

Oats

This grain is a blessing for chemotherapy patients. It's a comfort to start the day with a big bowl of warm oatmeal. Oats lowers cholesterol, boost the immune system, and contain special antioxidants called avenanthramides, which prevent free radicals from attacking good cholesterol and promote general good health for cancer recovery. Although oatmeal contains a small amount of gluten, studies have shown that oatmeal is well tolerated by both adults and children with celiac disease.

Eggs with Spinach and Tomato

1 egg, poached or soft-boiled
3 c. spinach, trimmed, coarsely chopped
1 tomato, chopped
1/8 c. water (for steaming)
Salt and pepper to taste

Place the water in a medium saucepan, and bring to a boil. Add the spinach and tomatoes. Cover and steam on medium heat for 2 minutes. Drain water and add seasoning. Serve hot over egg.

Serving: 1

Spinach

Flavonoids, a phytonutrient with anti-cancer properties abundant in spinach, slow down cell division in human stomach and skin cancer cells. Spinach also offers significant protection against the occurrence of aggressive prostate cancer. It has anti-inflammatory properties and is rich in the antioxidants vitamin C, vitamin E, beta-carotene, manganese, zinc, and selenium. One cup of spinach contains over 337% of the RDA of vitamin A, which protects and strengthens "entry points" into the human body—the mucous membranes, respiratory, urinary and intestinal tracts—and is also a key component of lymphocytes (or white blood cells) that fight infection.

Steel-Cut Oats with Walnuts and Apples

1 c. steel-cut oats
1 c. water
1 Granny Smith apple, chopped
1/8 c. walnuts, chopped

Soak oats in the water overnight, covering the oats completely. In the morning, add the chopped apple and cook over a medium to low heat for 3 minutes or until mixture reaches a hot temperature. Stir in walnuts. Serve warm.

Serving: 1

Walnuts

The wide variety of antioxidant and anti-inflammatory nutrients in walnuts makes them particularly beneficial for cancer patients. They help to lower the risk of chronic oxidative stress, and the anti-inflammatory properties help lower the risk of chronic inflammation—two types of risk, that, when combined, pose the greatest threat for cancer development. If buying walnuts in bulk, Dr. Oz says to keep walnuts refrigerated—otherwise they can get rancid

---

Buckwheat Porridge

2 c. buckwheat

3 c. water

1/2 c. almond milk or seed milk

1/2 c. raisins or chopped green apples

Pinch of sea salt

1-1/2 tsp. cinnamon

Soak buckwheat in the water overnight, covering the buckwheat completely. In the morning, rinse and drain the buckwheat thoroughly.

Add the buckwheat to a pan and cover it with water. Cook the buckwheat for 3-5 minutes or until soft, and add a pinch of salt.

Mix in cinnamon, almond milk, raisins or apple. Cook for 1-2 more minutes. Serve warm.

Servings: 2

Oat Waffles or Pancakes Topped with Almond Butter and Berries

2 c. rolled oats
1/8 c. raisins
1/4 c. almond milk (unsweetened)
1/4 c. water (to thin the mixture, if needed)
1/4 tsp. sea salt
1-2 tsps. coconut oil

Topping
1-3 Tbsps. almond butter
1-1/2 c. berries of your liking

In a blender, mix all the ingredients (except water and coconut oil) until smooth. Add water to thin the mixture if needed.

Lightly oil the waffle iron or pan with coconut oil. Pour or spoon out the mixture onto the cooking surface and cook until golden brown on each side.

Cover with the topping and serve.

Servings: 2

Warm Quinoa Cereal

1-1/2 c. quinoa, cooked, warm
1/2 tsp. coconut oil
Sea salt, pinch
Nutmeg, pinch
1/4 tsp. cinnamon
1/4 c. almonds, chopped
1 c. almond milk

Warm the quinoa in a medium saucepan with the coconut oil on a low heat. Add the spices. Stir constantly. Remove from heat and place in a cereal bowl. Top with the almonds and add milk.

Servings: 2

Notes

Notes

DRINKS

Ginger Tea

1 Tbsp. fresh ginger (or 1 tsp. powdered)

1 c. water

Peel and dice or grate the fresh ginger. In a pan, bring water to a boil and add the ginger. Cover and allow steeping for at least 5 minutes.

Serve hot or cold as iced tea.

Serving: 1

Ginger

Ginger is the great gift to chemotherapy patients because it goes directly to one of the most common side-effects of chemo—nausea and other digestive problems. One recent study shows ginger to be far superior to Dramamine, a commonly used over-the-counter and prescription drug for motion sickness. Ginger reduces all symptoms associated with motion sickness including dizziness, nausea, vomiting, and cold sweating.

Raw Almond Milk

1 c. raw almonds, soaked overnight
4-5 c. water
1 tsp. vanilla
Sea salt, pinch

Blend the almonds and half the water in a blender on a medium to low speed setting. Next, blend on high until consistency is smooth.

Add the rest of the water, salt, and pure vanilla extract. Blend again. Strain through a metal or plastic strainer—or cheesecloth for a smoother consistency.

Reserve the almond pulp for other recipes.

Chill and serve.

Servings: 4-5 cups

Brown Rice Milk

1/2 c. cooked brown rice
2 c. water
1 tsp. pure vanilla extract
Sea salt, pinch

Combine ingredients in a blender and mix until smooth. Strain through a metal or plastic strainer—or cheesecloth for a smoother consistency. Keep the milk and discard the rice pulp.

Servings: 2 cups

Oat Milk

1/2 c. uncooked oats, any kind except "instant" or "one-minute"
4 c. water at room temperature

Soak the oats in the water for 20 minutes. Soak directly in a blender, if you are short of time or if using fine-rolled oats. Blend. Strain for a smoother consistency. Refrigerated, oat milk lasts up to a week.

Servings: 4 cups

Green Lemonade

---

3 kale sprigs, washed

2 handfuls spinach, washed

1/2 cucumber, washed

1 lemon, peeled

1-1/2 green or red apples

1 inch ginger root, washed (or 1/2 tsp. of powdered ginger root)

With a juice extractor

Cut fruit, vegetables, and ginger so they fit in the juice extractor. Extract juice. Drink within 30 minutes for best nutritional benefits.

With a blender

Chop fruits and vegetables and place in a blender. Blend for 1 minute or slightly longer. Do not attempt to blend ginger root in an electric blender because it will get stuck in the blades. When using a blender, substitute ginger powder for ginger root.

Strain through a plastic or metal (non-aluminum) strainer. Mix with a spoon if the liquid is not flowing through the strainer. Discard or compost the pulp.

Serving: 1

Chai Rooibos

1/4-1/2 vanilla bean
10 cardamom seeds
5 whole cloves
1 ½ inch cinnamon stick
1 black peppercorn
Stevia to taste
Rooibos tea
4 c. water

Grind the spices in a spice grinder and add to a teapot. Add 3 heaping teaspoons of rooibos tea and 4 cups boiling water. Add stevia for extra sweetness, if desired, and steep for 10 minutes or longer. Also good iced.

Servings: 4 cups

Source: Laurel de Leo

Rooibos tea

The antioxidants in rooibos tea have been shown to increase the productivity of carcinogen-detoxifying enzymes, as well as protecting cell proteins, cell fats, and DNA. Its effective combination of antioxidants and important minerals gives the immune system a boost. For chemo patients, rooibos tea brings relief from stomach cramps. Rich in manganese, fluoride and calcium, rooibos tea promotes good bone growth during treatment.

Mean Green Juice #1

6 kale leaves

1 cucumber

4 celery stalks

2 green apples

1/2 lemon, peeled with some white rind left

1 tsp. powdered ginger

Combine all ingredients in a blender and mix well.

Serving: 1

Source: This and the three "Mean Green Juices" that follow are the official recipes used by Joe Cross and Phil Staples of the Reboot Your Life Program.

Celery

Celery contains compounds called coumarins. They help prevent free radicals from damaging cells by decreasing the mutations that increase the potential for cells to become cancerous. Coumarins also enhance the activity of certain white blood cells. In addition, compounds in celery called acetylenics have been shown to stop the growth of tumor cells.

Mean Green Juice #2

1 handful spinach

3 stalks kale

2 Golden Delicious apples

1 small handful parsley

1 lemon, peeled with some white rind

1 cucumber

Combine all ingredients in a blender and mix well.

Serving: 1

Mean Green Juice #3

2 stalks celery

1/2 cucumber

1/2 apple

1/2 lemon, peeled with some white rind left

1 tsp. powdered ginger

1/2 green chard leaf

1 small bunch cilantro

5 kale leaves

1 handful spinach

Combine all ingredients in a blender and mix well.

Serving: 1

Mean Green Juice #4

1/2 pear
1/2 green apple
1 handful spinach
1 small handful parsley
2 celery stalks
1/2 cucumber
1 tsp. powdered ginger, small piece
1 slice papaya

Combine all ingredients in a blender and mix well.

Serving: 1

Blueberry Smoothie

1 c. blueberries (fresh or frozen)
1 c. oat milk (see recipe on page 119)
3 or 6 ice cubes

Add all ingredients in a blender and mix until smooth. If using fresh blueberries, add 3 more ice cubes for a thinner consistency.

Serving: 1

Blueberries

Blueberries are nutritional superstars. These fruits contain significant amounts of anthocyanins, anti-oxidant compounds that give blue, purple and red colors to fruits and vegetables. In addition to their anthocyanins, blueberries are an excellent source of bone-healthy vitamin K and a good source of free-radical-scavenging vitamin C and manganese. Blueberries also provide a generous amount of fiber for a healthy heart and help in detoxing.

Strawberry Walnut Smoothie

1 c. strawberries (fresh or frozen)
1 c. milk (oat, rice, almond, or seed)
10 walnut halves
3-6 ice cubes

Place all ingredients in the blender and mix on a medium to high speed for 1-2 minutes. Adjust the consistency with more milk or ice cubes.

Serving: 1

Lemon / Lime Water

1 lemon or lime, juiced

4 c. cold water

8-10 ice cubes (optional)

In a large water pitcher add all ingredients and stir. This is refreshing to sip on through the day, and an excellent liver detox.

Servings: 4

Cucumber Water

3 cucumber slices

4 c. water

8-10 ice cubes (optional)

Add all ingredients to a large pitcher and serve.

Servings: 4

Cucumber

Cucumbers have valuable antioxidant, anti-inflammatory, and anti-cancer properties. Substances in fresh cucumber extracts help scavenge free radicals, help improve antioxidant status, inhibit the activity of pro-inflammatory enzymes, and prevent overproduction of nitric oxide in situations where it could pose health risks.

Rooibos Ice Tea

2-3 Tbsps. rooibos tea leaves in a tea ball or use 4 tea bags

3 c. water

5-10 ice cubes

Heat water and tea leaves in a large sauce pan over medium-high heat. When the water boils, cover, turn down the heat and simmer for 10-15 minutes. Cool 30 minutes and pour over ice.

Servings: 3

Green Tea

2-3 Tbsps. green tea in a tea ball
5 c. water

Bring water to a boil and turn off the heat. Add the tea ball and cover for 3-5 minutes or longer for stronger tea. Drink hot or over ice.

Servings: 4

Green Tea

Green tea has been called the "miracle tea," and has been used in China for its considerable health benefits for over 4000 years. Research shows that regular green tea drinkers do not contract common bacterial and viral infections easily. Green tea boosts immunity. It has been used for many years to treat cancer, rheumatoid arthritis, high cholesterol levels, cardiovascular disease, infection, and impaired immune function.

Ginger, Strawberry, Green Tea Smoothie

1 c. green tea

3-5 strawberries, fresh or frozen, trimmed

1/2 c. almond milk or oat milk

1/2 tsp. ginger powder

2-5 ice cubes

Add all ingredients in a blender, mix on medium speed for 1-3 minutes or until the mixture is smooth.

Servings: 2

Green Drink Smoothie

1 c. green tea
1/2 avocado, peeled and pitted
1/2 tsp. or more spirulina
1/2 tsp. ginger powder
2 ice cubes

Combine all ingredients in a blender. Mix on a high speed until it is smooth and creamy.

Servings: 2

Oatmeal Blackberry Smoothie

1/2 c. blackberries, frozen or fresh
1/2 c. oatmeal, cooked
1-1/2 c. rooibos tea

Combine all ingredients in a blender. Mix on a high speed until smooth and creamy.

Servings: 2

Notes

Notes

SOUPS

Spiced Split-Pea Soup

2 c. dried split-peas
8 c. boiling water
1 medium-sized onion
3 (or more) cloves garlic, chopped
2 zucchini, chopped
1/2 c. chopped parsley
1 tsp. chili powder or one fresh pepper

Bring water to a boil. In a large soup pot, add split-peas to boiling water and cook for about 30-45 minutes, or until the split-peas are tender. Add the remaining ingredients and continue cooking until the vegetables are tender. Add more water to adjust the consistency, if desired.

Servings: 3

Onions

The health benefits of onions are so many and various they would practically fill their own book. For cancer patients, the onion's anti-inflammatory qualities are amazing. Onions are excellent, also, for cardiovascular function and for general health. Inexpensive, onions are worth their weight in gold.

Fresh Tomato Soup

1 large onion, chopped
5 small ripe tomatoes, chopped
1-1/2 c. water
1 tsp. parsley flakes or equivalent fresh
Dash of pepper and salt

Combine all ingredients in a large pot. Cook over medium heat for 15 minutes. Cool a few minutes. Blend in blender, reheat, and serve.

Servings: 2

Source: *chooseveg.com*

Tomatoes

Various studies have shown that because of the high lycopene content in tomatoes, the red fruit (yes, it's technically a fruit) helps to lessen the chances of prostate cancer in men, and reduces the chance of stomach cancer and colorectal cancer. Lycopene is considered a natural miracle antioxidant that may help to stop the growth of cancer cells. Cooked tomatoes produce more lycopene than do raw tomatoes.

Mushroom Barley Soup

2 c. rice milk

2 Tbsps. barley flour

1 c. cooked barley

2 c. mushrooms (shiitake, Portobello, oyster), chopped

1-2 cloves of garlic, chopped fine

1/4 tsp. sea salt or pink salt

Pinch each of dried marjoram, sage, thyme, and dill weed

Place rice milk and barley flour in a blender. Blend on high speed for a few seconds. Add barley and blend on high for about 10 seconds, or until barley is coarsely chopped.

Add mushrooms with their liquid. Blend just enough to coarsely chop mushrooms.

Transfer the blended mixture to a medium-sized saucepan and add all the remaining ingredients. Cook over medium heat, stirring often, for about 5 minutes, or until the soup is hot and somewhat thickened.

Servings: 2

Source: **Foods That Fight Pain** *by Neal Barnard, M.D. (New York: Random House, 1999), recipe by Jennifer Raymond, M.S., R.D.*

Mushrooms

Mushrooms are an excellent source of potassium, a mineral that helps lower elevated blood pressure and reduces the risk of stroke. One medium Portobello mushroom has even more potassium than a banana or a glass of orange juice. Shiitake mushrooms have been used for centuries by the Chinese and Japanese to treat colds and flu. Lentinan, taken from the fruiting body of shiitake mushrooms, stimulates the immune system, helps fight infection, and demonstrates anti-tumor activity.

Winter Squash and Red Lentil Stew

1 c. red lentils or yellow split-peas
3-1/2 c. water
1 onion, chopped
1/2 tsp. each mustard seeds, turmeric, ginger, and cumin
1/4 tsp. cinnamon
1/8 tsp. cayenne
4 c. peeled and diced winter squash (about 2 pounds)
1 Tbsp. lemon juice
1/2 tsp. salt or to taste

Place the lentils and 2 cups water in a pot and bring to a simmer. Cover loosely and cook until the lentils are tender, about 20 minutes.

Braise the onion in 1/2 cup water until soft and translucent, then add the spices, the remaining 1-1/2 cups water, and the diced squash. Cover and cook over medium heat until the squash is tender when pierced with a fork, about 15 minutes. Stir in the lemon juice, cooked lentils, and salt to taste.

Servings: 3

Source: chooseveg.com

Butternut Squash and Apple Soup

1 butternut squash, chopped
2 or more garlic cloves, chopped
2 green apples, peeled and chopped
4 c. vegetable stock
Salt and pepper to taste
Cayenne pepper garnish

In a large frying pan, steam the squash, apples, and garlic together with about 2 cups of the vegetable stock for 10-15 minutes, covered. When the squash, apples, and garlic are cooked to a nice softness, let cool for a few minutes and transfer to a blender and slowly add the remaining two cups of stock until soup is smooth. Serve hot. Garnish with a dash of cayenne pepper.

Servings: 4

Source: *adapted from chooseveg.com*

Barley Vegetable Soup

2 Tbsps. olive oil

2 onions, peeled and chopped

2 carrots, diced

2 stalks celery, chopped

8 c. water

3 large tomatoes, chopped

1 tsp. salt

1 tsp. dried basil

1/2 tsp. dried thyme

1/2 tsp. black pepper

1 c. pearl barley

2 c. green beans, chopped

2 Tbsps. fresh dill, chopped

In a large pot, heat olive oil over a medium heat. Add onions, carrots and celery, and sauté until softened. Add water, tomatoes, salt, basil, thyme, and pepper; bring to a boil.

Stir in barley. Lower heat and cover. Gently simmer for 1-1/2 hours or until barley is tender. Stir in fresh green beans during the last 10 minutes of cooking. Remove from heat and stir in dill weed. Serve warm.

Servings: 4

Healthy Bean Soup with Kale

1 Tbsp. olive oil

8 garlic cloves, minced

1 medium yellow onion, chopped

4 c. raw kale, deveined, chopped

4 c. vegetable broth, divided

3 c. cooked beans (black beans, pinto, white beans, lentils, or mix and match beans together)

5 tomatoes, diced

2 tsps. Italian herb seasoning

1 c. chopped parsley

Salt and pepper to taste

In a large pot, heat olive oil, and add garlic and onion. Sauté until soft and the onion is transparent. Wash the kale, leaving small droplets of water. Sauté, stirring, until wilted and a lovely emerald green, about 15 minutes. Add 3 cups of the broth, 2 cups of the beans, all of the carrots, tomatoes, herbs, salt and pepper.

Simmer 5 minutes. In a blender or food processor, mix the reserved 1 cup of beans and 1 cup of broth until smooth. Stir into the soup to thicken it nicely. Simmer 15 more minutes. Serve warm, garnished with parsley.

Servings: 8

Source: food.com

White Bean, Squash and Kale Soup

1 pound dried white beans	8 c. water
2 onions, coarsely chopped	1 tsp. salt
2 Tbsps. olive oil	1 bay leaf
4 garlic cloves, minced	5 c. vegetable stock
1/2 tsp. black pepper	1 tsp. rosemary, chopped fine
1/2 butternut squash, peeled, seeded and cut into 1/2-inch cubes	1 pound kale, deveined, chopped

Soak beans for at least 8 hours, changing the water several times. Then simmer the beans in enough water to cover them for about 30 minutes, or until they are about halfway to tender.

Sauté onions in oil in a large pot over medium-low heat until softened, 4-5 minutes. Add garlic and cook, stirring, 1 minute. Add beans, stock, 4 cups water, salt, pepper, bay leaf, and rosemary and simmer uncovered about 20 minutes. Add the squash and simmer another 30 minutes until beans and squash are tender. Stir in kale and the remaining 4 cups of water and simmer uncovered, until kale is tender, 12 to 15 minutes. Season soup with salt and pepper and serve.   Servings: 6

Source: Jen Klien – sheknows.com, adapted by Dr. Mike

Vegan Irish Stew

4 c. veggie broth

2-3 c. green beans, cleaned and ends trimmed, cut into 1" pieces

2 c. cashews

2 c. cooked brown rice (or your favorite rice/rice mix - mine consists of 1/2 brown rice, 1/4 wild rice, and 1/4 lentils)

1/2 c. sauerkraut with juice

1/2 c. nutritional yeast

1 Tbsp. Bragg's Liquid Aminos

1 tsp. lemon juice

1 tsp. dill weed

Salt and pepper to taste

Bring vegetable broth to a boil. Add green beans, cover, lower heat and simmer for 10 minutes. Place a colander over a large bowl and drain the beans, reserving the veggie broth. Add veggie broth to a blender along with the cashews and process until completely smooth.

Pour broth/cashew mix back into pot, along with green beans and remaining ingredients. Heat over low flame until warmed.

Servings: 4-6

Source: Patty "Sassy" Knutson – vegancoach.com

Hearty Vegan Vegetable Soup

8 c. vegetable broth
1/2 c. uncooked barley
4 tomatoes, chopped
1 large onion
3 celery stalks
4 large carrots, unpeeled and sliced
3 large red potatoes, unpeeled and chunked
1 tsp. each basil, rosemary, celery seeds
1 tsp. lemon juice
Sea salt and pepper to taste

Place vegetable broth in a large pot and bring to a simmer. Add barley and cook while prepping the rest of the veggies. Add the tomatoes, onion, celery, and potatoes. Continue to boil for 40 minutes.

When veggies and barley are tender, stir in basil, rosemary, celery seeds. Remove from heat. While cooling, add lemon juice. Season to taste with salt and pepper.

Servings: 6

Source: Patty "Sassy" Knutson – vegancoach.com

Barley

Barley is rich in phosphorus, which is important to the development and repair of body tissue. Phosphorus is a vital component of nucleic acids, the building blocks of the genetic code. A cup of cooked barley gives us 23% of the daily value for phosphorus.

Vegetable Bean Soup

1 c. carrots, diced

1 c. zucchini, diced

3/4 c. onion, chopped

1/2 c. chopped sweet red pepper

1 Tbsp. olive oil

2 c. vegetable broth

1 c. kidney beans, cooked

1 c. garbanzo beans, cooked

3-4 fresh tomatoes, skinned, chopped

4 tsps. ground cumin

1/4 tsp. cayenne pepper

2 Tbsps. fresh cilantro, minced

In a large saucepan or Dutch oven, sauté the carrots, zucchini, onion, tomatoes, and red pepper in oil until crisp-tender. Add the broth, beans, cumin and cayenne; bring to a boil.

Reduce heat; simmer, uncovered, for 30-35 minutes or until vegetables are tender, stirring occasionally. At the end, stir in cilantro.

Servings: 4-6

Zucchini

Because dietary fiber promotes healthy and regular bowel movements, the high amounts of fiber in zucchini also help prevent carcinogenic toxins from settling in the colon. Moreover, the vitamins C and A, as well as folate, found in zucchini act as powerful antioxidants that fight oxidative stress that can lead to many different types of cancer. The vitamins C and A in zucchini not only serve the body as powerful antioxidants, but also as effective anti-inflammatory agents.

Notes

Notes

MAIN DISHES

Black Bean and Zucchini Tortilla Casserole

1-1/2 tsps. extra virgin olive oil

1 c. onion

2 garlic cloves, finely chopped

1 medium red or yellow pepper

3 tomatoes

1-3 small fresh chili peppers, seeded and minced

2 tsps. chili powder, to taste

1 tsp. dried oregano

1 tsp. ground cumin

1 tsp. turmeric powder

2 c. black beans, cooked and drained

2 medium zucchinis, chopped thin

12 corn tortillas, torn or cut into several pieces

1 egg, whisked

Preheat the oven to 400 degrees. Heat the oil in a large saucepan. Sauté onion until translucent. Add the red or yellow pepper and continue to sauté until it has softened and the onions are golden.

Stir in the tomatoes and seasonings, black beans, and zucchini. Over medium heat, simmer gently for 5 minutes. Add the tortillas and egg with the cooked bean and veggie mix. Mix well and place in a 9 x 13 inch or two quart round casserole dish.

Bake for 15-20 minutes and let cool and set for 5 minutes. Spoon and serve warm.

Servings: 3-4

Source: Adapted from **The Vegetarian Family Cookbook** *by Nava Atlas (New York: Clarkson Potter, 2004)*

Classic Caesar Salad with Shrimp

1-1/2 pounds of uncooked
large shrimp (24-28), peeled
and deveined
1 tsp. sea salt
1 head romaine lettuce
1/2 c. parmesan cheese
4 oil-packed anchovy fillets

Caesar Dressing
1/4 c. parmesan cheese, grated
4 anchovy fillets
2 egg yolks
1/4 tsp. salt, to taste
1/4 tsp. pepper, to taste
1 lemon, juice and zest
1/2 c. extra virgin olive oil
2 garlic cloves

Remove outer leaves of romaine lettuce, wash and dry inner leaves, tear into halves.

Fill a large pot with water. Bring to a boil over a medium-high heat. Add the shrimp and salt. Cook until the shrimp are opaque, about 2-3 minutes. Pull a shrimp from the pot, cut into the center to check that the shrimp is completely opaque. Drain the shrimp. Place in cold water to stop the cooking process. Dry the shrimp.

Prepare the dressing: In blender, mix egg yolks, garlic, and anchovies into a paste. Add remaining ingredients except olive oil. Mix a few seconds. Slowly add olive oil until dressing is thick and creamy. Add more or less olive oil depending on desired consistency.

In a large salad bowl, toss the romaine with the dressing. Add half of the parmesan cheese. Toss again. Place the salad on four dinner plates. Distribute the shrimp evenly over greens. Sprinkle with the remaining parmesan. Place an anchovy in the middle of each salad. Serve.

Servings: 4

Source: Jessica Strand, from her book Salad Dressings *(San Francisco: Chronicle Books, 2007)*

Fish Tacos

4 tilapia fillets

1/4 red onion, thinly sliced

2 Tbsps. coconut oil

1/2 tsp. cumin powder

1/2 tsp. dried oregano

2 limes, cut in half

8 corn tortillas

8 Tbsp. Garden Fresh Salsa
  (see recipe on page 192)

Pre-heat a gas grill on medium heat. In a large bowl, mix the coconut oil and spices together well. Place the fish in the bowl and carefully coat on all sides, or use a grilling brush. Place the fish on the hot grill and cook for about 2 minutes each side. Remove one fillet and cut lengthwise right down the center to check for a white flaky consistency. Warm corn tortillas on the grill.

Assemble the taco: start with a warm soft tortilla, add strips of fish, slivered onion, Garden Fresh Salsa, and a squeeze of lime. Serve with a green salad or sprouts.

Servings: 4

Garbanzo Beans with Ginger and Tomatoes

1 onion, chopped

4 tomatoes, chopped

2 c. garbanzo beans, cooked

1 Tbsp. extra virgin olive oil

2 Tbsps. ginger, grated

1/4 tsp. turmeric

1 tsp. cumin

1 tsp. cinnamon

2 Tbsps. cilantro, chopped

Salt and pepper to taste

Sauté onions, ginger, and tomatoes in oil until tomatoes are juicy, about 10 minutes. Add garbanzo beans and spices. Stir and simmer for 5-10 minutes to blend flavors. Season to taste with salt and pepper. Garnish with cilantro.

Servings: 4

Source: Vegan Dinner Recipes – vegkitchen.com

Garbanzo beans (Chickpeas)

Chemo patients will find garbanzo beans an excellent source of fiber, which is useful in forcing toxins out of the body. Garbanzos offer a good supply of magnesium and folic acid. Also found in garbanzo beans is molybdenum, a trace mineral needed for the body's mechanism to detoxify sulfites, a preservative commonly found in wine and luncheon meats.

Swiss Chard with Garbanzo Beans and Fresh Tomatoes

2 Tbsp. olive oil

1 shallot, chopped

2 green onions, chopped

1/2 c. garbanzo beans, cooked

1 bunch red Swiss chard, rinsed and chopped

1 tomato, chopped

1/2 lemon, juice

Sea salt, to taste

Black pepper, to taste

Heat olive oil in a large skillet. Stir in shallot and green onions; cook and stir for 3-5 minutes, or until soft and fragrant. Stir in garbanzo beans, and season with salt and pepper; heat through. Place chard in pan, and cook until wilted. Add tomato, squeeze lemon juice over greens, and heat through. Plate, and season with salt and pepper to taste.

Servings: 2

Asparagus and Mushroom Quinoa Risotto

4 c. vegetable broth
1 c. sliced mushrooms
1 c. dry quinoa
1 bunch asparagus
Salt to taste

1 small yellow or white onion
1 Tbsp. olive oil
2 Tbsps. lemon juice
1 Tbsp. plant-based buttery spread such as Earth Balance or Better-Than-Butter Garlic spread, page 200

Start by pouring the vegetable broth into a saucepan and bringing it up to a light simmer. Having hot stock or broth is an important step in making risotto. Next, dice the onion and mushrooms and sauté in olive oil over medium heat. This is one instance where you definitely want to use stainless cookware rather than something non-stick. You want the onions and mushrooms to create some browning on the bottom of the pan.

Once the onion and mushroom are browning, add the dry quinoa and stir to coat in the olive oil. Continue to stir and cook over medium high heat for about 3 minutes – just enough to coat the quinoa and toast it a bit.

Add 2 tablespoons of lemon juice to deglaze the bottom of the pan, and then begin adding the hot vegetable stock to the quinoa one ladle at a time.

Add stock and stir continuously over medium heat until most liquid is absorbed. Once absorbed, add another ladle full of stock, and continue to do so for 25-30 minutes total, or until quinoa is cooked and risotto is creamy. In between ladles and stirring, cut asparagus into bite-sized pieces. Make sure to trim the woody ends! When you only have 3 or 4 ladles left, add the raw asparagus to your mixture and stir to combine and cook. Continue to cook and stir until almost all liquid is absorbed. Finish by adding 1 tablespoon Earth Balance for a touch more creaminess, and season to taste with salt.

Servings: 4

Shiitake Mushroom Salad

4 oz. shiitake mushrooms, trimmed and sliced

1 1/2 tsp. olive oil

4-5 c. mixed greens

1/2 c. green beans, cut in thin strips

1/3 c. carrots, cut in thin strips

1/3 c. red bell pepper, cut thin

3 Tbsps. walnuts, chopped

Dressing

1 Tbsp. red wine vinegar or apple cider vinegar

3 Tbsps. olive oil

1 clove garlic, crushed

Salt and pepper to taste

Sauté shiitake mushrooms in 1 1/2 olive oil over medium heat until browned. Remove from the heat and set aside covered to steam.

To make dressing, combine vinegar, garlic, salt and pepper and slowly add olive oil.

In a medium bowl, add beans, nuts, carrots, mushrooms, and red pepper with dressing to coat. Toss with lettuce. Serve.

Servings: 4

Carrots

Carrots are an outstanding source of the phytonutrient (antioxidant, immune boosting and other health-promoting) properties beta-carotene. In addition, carrots are an excellent source of vitamin A and of immune-supportive vitamin C, bone-building vitamin K, and heart-healthy dietary fiber, and potassium.

Rice Noodles with Asparagus

6 oz. rice sticks or rice vermicelli

2 tsps. toasted sesame oil, divided

2 large eggs (optional)

1/4 tsp. white or black pepper

2 c. asparagus, trimmed and chopped into bite-sized pieces

2 c. snow peas, trimmed and sliced lengthwise

3 cloves garlic, minced

3/4 c. vegetable broth

2 tsp. sriracha sauce or chili oil (optional)

3 green onions, thinly sliced

Soak rice sticks in large bowl of hot water 8 minutes. Drain well. In a large frying pan on a medium-high heat, add 1 tsp. of sesame oil and add two eggs, water, and pepper. Mix the eggs while they cook to a soft scramble. Cover and set aside. In a wok or large frying pan, stir-fry in the sesame oil the asparagus, snow peas, and garlic for 3-5 minutes on a medium heat. Add sriracha or chili oil to steam. Let the liquid be absorbed.

Add the cooked eggs, green onion, and rice noodles. Mix. Cover for one minute and serve.

Servings: 4

Snow peas

Snow peas are extremely healthy to add to dishes and to munch on, because the potent healthy nutrients in them are tremendously nourishing. The nutrients in snow peas are fiber, carbohydrates, protein, vitamins A and C, healthy fats, iron, potassium, magnesium, folic acid, and antioxidants. These nutrients have the ability to relieve and prevent inflammation, cancers, eye diseases, and digestive issues.

Grilled Sardines

8-10 whole sardines, fresh or frozen, cleaned (organs removed)

Dry rub mix

1 tsp. garlic powder

3/4 tsp. turmeric

1 tsp. salt

1 tsp. cornstarch

1/2 tsp. cayenne pepper

1/2 tsp. black pepper

Sauce

3 Tbsps. coconut oil

1 Tbsp. coconut milk

1/4 c. fresh coriander, chopped

2 Tbsps. vegetable stock

3-4 Tbsps. lime juice

2 cloves garlic minced

Lightly oil the grill with a little cooking oil to prevent fish from sticking.

To make the barbecue dry rub, simply stir all rub ingredients together in a small bowl. If the sardines are already cleaned and prepared, skip this step. If not, make a cut along the bottom of the fish and remove the intestines and entrails (simply run your finger inside the cut). Rinse and place the fish aside to dry.

Place prepared sardines on a tray or in a long casserole dish, so that they're lying flat. Drizzle 1 Tbsp. vegetable oil and spread evenly over the fish. Sprinkle the barbecue dry rub over the entire surface of the fish. Gently rub along each fish, so they appear yellow-gold. Sprinkle any remaining rub powder over the fish and set aside to marinate until grill is hot (at least 10 minutes).

To make the sauce: Place ingredients in a small pot or saucepan. Warm up over medium heat to bring out the flavors. Season to taste.

Grill the fish until cooked, about 5-8 minutes each side. When done, the fish will appear golden and the skin will be crisp.

Servings: 4

Shrimp and Spinach Salad

2 Tbsps. almond milk

2 Tbsps. olive oil

1 lemon juice and zest

10 oz. spinach leaves, cleaned

12 oz. medium shrimp, poached

1/2 red onion, diced

1 Granny Smith apple, peeled, seeded and diced

1/3 c. walnut pieces

1/4 c. parsley, chopped

Salt and pepper to taste

Whisk almond milk and olive oil, the juice and finely grated zest of 1 lemon, salt and pepper to taste. Toss together spinach, shrimp, red onion, apple, walnuts and parsley.

Servings: 3

Avocado and Shrimp Salad

1 lb. cooked shrimp, deveined, shelled and cubed

1 large avocado, ripe

Mixed spring greens

3 Tbsps. olive oil

2 Tbsps. white wine vinegar

1 tsp. Dijon mustard

1/2 lemon juice

1 Tbsp. chili sauce

1/2 garlic clove, minced

2 Tbsp. fresh dill, finely minced

2 Tbsp. fresh chives, finely minced

Salt and pepper to taste

In a large bowl whisk together all ingredients except shrimp, avocado, and spring greens. Add shrimp and avocado, toss lightly. Season to taste. Cover and chill until ready to serve. Serve on bed of mixed spring greens.

Servings: 4

Grilled Salmon Salad

4 medium to small salmon steaks
1 Tbsp. organic coconut oil
1 tsp. lemon juice
1 tsp. dill (fresh or dried)
Fresh ground black pepper
1 bag of organic mixed greens
Dressing
5 strawberries, trimmed
2 Tbsp. olive oil
1-3 splashes of Tabasco sauce or other hot sauce

In a large bowl, combine olive oil, lemon juice, dill, black pepper and Tabasco. Mix well. Coat the salmon in the mixture and grill on a medium flame or oven bake at 350 degrees for 15 minutes or until the centers are cooked throughout.

Make the dressing by combining ingredients in a blender, and mix well. Add water to thin or extra strawberry to thicken.

In a large bowl, add the salad greens and dressing. Toss gently to evenly coat the greens. Top with cooked salmon.

Servings: 4

Steamed Veggies with Black Bean Sauce

2 medium broccoli crowns, chopped

1 onion, chopped

30 green beans, trimmed and chopped

3 zucchini, chopped

1 c. water

Bean Sauce

1 c. cooked black beans

1/2 c. water or vegetable stock

1/2 garlic clove, peeled and chopped

1/2 tsp. cumin, powder

Salt and pepper to taste

In a large frying pan add broccoli, onions, and water. Cover and steam over medium heat for 4 minutes or until broccoli is a brilliant green color. Add green beans and zucchini. Cover, turn off the heat and let stand for 3-4 minutes.

Add all ingredients for the bean sauce in a blender. Mix till smooth. Water or vegetable stock may be added to thin the sauce. Drain the steamed vegetables and top with the bean sauce. Toss gently. Serve warm.

Servings: 4

Cumin

A natural antioxidant that helps fight cancer of the liver, improves digestion, and strengthens the immune system. In one study, cumin was shown to protect laboratory animals from developing stomach or liver tumors. This cancer-protective effect may be due to cumin's potent free radical scavenging abilities as well as the ability it has shown to enhance the liver's detoxification enzymes.

Black Bean Veggie Chili

2 medium onions, chopped
4 garlic cloves, minced
1-1/2 c. bean sprouts
2 c. black beans, cooked
5 medium tomatoes
2 medium zucchini
1/2 c. dried chipotle chili peppers (remove seeds)
2 tsps. cumin
2 tsps. turmeric
1 Tbsp. extra virgin olive oil
Salt and pepper to taste
Avocado slices

Lightly sauté the onions and garlic in the olive oil. Add tomatoes and zucchini, and cook for 20 minutes, stirring occasionally. Add beans, chili peppers and spices and cook another 5 minutes. Stir in bean sprouts, salt, and pepper. Garnish with avocado slices. Serve with corn tortillas.

Servings: 4-5

Chipotle chili

Chili peppers contain capsaicin, which gives them their characteristic pungency. The World Health Organization reports that in countries where diets are traditionally high in capsaicin, the cancer death rates are significantly lower than in countries with less chili pepper consumption. Capsaicin has been found to preferentially inhibit the growth of cancer cells in laboratory studies.

Shrimp Stir-Fry

10 medium-sized shrimp, peeled and deveined

1-2 yellow zucchini squash, sliced

1-2 broccoli crowns, chopped

1 c. bean sprouts

1 medium onion, chopped

1 c. jicama, chopped

1 c. snow peas

1/2 c. black beans, cooked (optional)

1 stalk celery, chopped

2 Tbsps. fresh ginger root, minced

Cayenne pepper to taste

1 c. water

In a wok or large saucepan, add water and bring to a boil. Add the vegetables one at a time, stirring along the way. Cook 5 minutes, until the vegetables are tender. Add the shrimp and allow to steam-cook for 5 more minutes. Add ginger and cayenne pepper.

Serve over curry rice, brown rice, or rice noodles.

Servings: 2-3

Shrimp

Shrimp is a rich source of the trace mineral selenium. Selenium helps in neutralizing the effects of free radicals, which are associated with cancer and other degenerative diseases. It is an excellent source of low-fat protein; around 23.7 grams of protein is gained from a 4 oz. serving of shrimp. Its anti-inflammatory properties aid in cancer recovery. Omega 3 fatty acids in shrimp also help slow down the development of cancerous tumors.

Fish Tacos with Cabbage Slaw

12 small corn tortillas

3 Tbsp. olive oil

3 Tbsp. lime juice

1/2 c. fresh cilantro, chopped

2-3 c. thinly sliced cabbage, mix of red and white varieties

3 green onions sliced thinly

1 small red onion sliced thinly

1 large tomato, chopped

1 lb. Tilapia fish fillets

3 cloves garlic, minced

1 tsp. ground cumin

1/4 tsp. each salt and freshly ground pepper

Olive oil cooking spray

6 lime wedges for garnish

Hot sauce (optional)

Preheat the oven to 300 degrees.

Place tortillas on a cookie sheet. When oven has reached correct temperature, place tortillas inside to warm. (This also could be done on grill while fish is cooking.)

To make the slaw, combine 2 Tbsps. oil, 2 Tbsps. lime juice, 1/4 cup cilantro, cabbage, green onions, red onion, and diced tomato in a bowl and set aside.

Season fish with garlic, cumin, salt, pepper, remaining oil and cilantro, and 1 Tbsp. lime juice. Heat grill or grill pan over medium-high heat. Spray with cooking oil spray. Place fish on grill/pan, careful to only turn once so it doesn't break apart. Let cook over medium high heat for about 4 minutes on first side and then about 2 minutes on second side. Let rest on large plate for about 5 minutes. Carefully flake apart the fish into roughly 1 inch size pieces.

Assemble tacos by placing fish and then slaw in each tortilla. Serve immediately with lime wedges and hot sauce, if desired.

Servings: 6

Source: American Institute for Cancer Research (http://www.aicr.org)

Autumn Stew

1-1/2 c. water or vegetable stock

1 onion, chopped

1 red bell pepper, diced

4 large garlic cloves, minced

1 lb. (about 4 c.) kabocha squash
  or other winter squash

3 tomatoes, chopped

1 1/2 tsps. chili powder

1/2 tsp. cumin

1/4 tsp. black pepper

1 c. cooked kidney beans

1 1/2 c. fresh or frozen corn

Heat 1/2 cup water in a large pot, then add the onion, bell pepper, and garlic. Cook over medium heat until the onion is translucent and most of the water evaporates.

Cut the squash in half and remove its seeds, then peel and cut it into half inch cubes. Add squash cubes to the onion mixture, along with the chopped tomatoes, remaining 1 cup water, oregano, chili powder, cumin, and pepper.

Cover and simmer until the squash is just tender when pierced with a fork, or about 20 minutes, then add the kidney beans with their liquid and the corn. Cook 5 minutes longer.

Servings: 5-6

Source: adapted from chooseveg.com

Kidney beans

Manganese, in which kidney beans are abundant, is one of the antioxidants they provide. The vitamin K in kidney beans has been shown to protect cells from oxidative stress, helping to heal from cancer. In addition, the vitamin K content offers outstanding benefits for the brain and nervous system. Kidney beans are also a good source of thiamin, which is critical for brain cell and cognitive function.

Notes

Notes

SIDE DISHES

Guacamole

3 ripe avocados - peeled, pitted, and mashed

1 lime, juiced

1 tsp. salt

1/2 c. onion, diced

3 Tbsps. fresh cilantro, chopped

1/4 tsp. ground cumin

2 plum (Roma) tomatoes, diced

1 tsp. minced garlic

1 pinch cayenne pepper (optional)

In a medium bowl, mash together the avocados, lime juice, and salt. Mix in onion, cilantro, tomatoes, cumin, and garlic. Stir in cayenne pepper. Refrigerate for an hour for best flavor, or serve immediately.

Servings: 4

Avocado

Avocado is rich in essential fatty acids, an enormous health benefit for people on chemo. It is also an excellent source of fiber, potassium, and several other vitamins, including B6 and C. High in antioxidant and anti-inflammatory values. Research is showing that avocado will selectively aid in the destruction of cancer cells, while supporting non-cancerous cells.

Curry Brown Rice

1 c. brown rice, short or long-grain
1-1/2 c. water
1 tsp. curry powder
1 Tbsp. brown raisins (optional)

Stir in curry powder and raisins, cover and let simmer for another 10 minutes.

Turn off the heat and, with the lid on, allow the rice to sit for another 10 minutes.

NOTE: this is a dish you can make ahead of time in quantity and keep in the refrigerator. To serve hot the next day, bring ½ cup of water to a boil and add the cold rice.

Servings: 4

Curry powder

Turmeric, one of the main ingredients in curry powder, reduces the risk of developing prostate, breast, skin and colorectal cancer—possibly because of its antioxidant properties. It may also reduce the speed at which these cancers progress. Other ingredients in curry, such as chili pepper and even curcumin, are beneficial in boosting immunity.

Braised Fennel Recipe

2 large fennel bulbs

2 Tbsps. olive oil

1 tsp. sea or pink salt

1/2 tsp. anise powder

1/2 c. vegetable stock

2 Tbsps. chopped fennel fronds

Zest from 1 orange

1/2 lemon or lime, juiced

Cut the tops off the fennel bulbs, chop 2 tablespoons of the fronds and set aside. Slice the fennel bulbs in half, lengthwise, through the core. Slice each half lengthwise into quarters (you should get eight pieces total out of each fennel bulb), leaving some of the core attached so the pieces don't fall apart as they cook. In a large sauté pan over medium-high heat and place the fennel pieces in the pan in a single layer.

Reduce the heat to medium and cook the fennel pieces, without moving them, for at least 2 minutes. Sprinkle the salt over the fennel. Cook for a few minutes on each side (the trick is to keep them from separating . . . good luck!) Add the stock and anise. Bring the liquid to a boil, then reduce the heat down to low, cover the pan and simmer for 5 minutes. Top with zest and a splash of lemon (or lime) juice. Cover to steam for a 2 minutes. Serve warm.

Servings: 4

Source: simplyrecipes.com

Steamed Cabbage with Caraway

One head cabbage (red or green), chopped
3 Tbsps. extra virgin olive oil
1 tsp. caraway seeds
1/2 tsp. celery seeds
1-1/2 tsps. salt
1/2 tsp. black pepper

In a large soup pot, bring water and salt to a boil. Add the cabbage. Cook for 90 seconds and drain off the water. Return the cabbage to the large soup pot. Add olive oil, caraway seeds, celery seeds, and black pepper. Add salt to taste. Mix and serve warm.

Servings: 4-6

Ginger and Sesame Broccoli

1 Tbsp. sesame seeds

1/2 c. vegetable stock

1 Tbsp. dark sesame oil

1 Tbsp. organic coconut oil

1 pound broccoli florets, chopped

2-3 cloves of garlic, chopped fine

1 Tbsp. fresh ginger, chopped fine

Add the stock and dark sesame oil together in a small bowl, set aside. In a large frying pan with lid, melt coconut oil over a medium heat. Add the broccoli florets, sauté and stir for about a minute. Mix in the ginger and garlic. Add the vegetable stock mixture to the pan. Bring to a simmer, reduce the heat and cover. Let cook for 2-3 minutes, until broccoli is tender and bright green. Garnish with sesame seeds.

Servings: 4

Source: simplyrecipes.com

Broccoli

The combination of antioxidant, anti-inflammatory, and pro-detoxification components in broccoli make it a unique food for the prevention of cancer. New research has made it clear that our risk of cancer in several different organ systems is related to the combination of these three problems. The rich nutrients found in broccoli directly address inflammation, oxidative stress, and detoxification.

Chayote with Tomato and Green Chili Recipe

3 chayotes, peeled and chopped

3 tomatoes, chopped

2 clove garlic, chopped fine

1 Tbsp. olive oil

1/2 red or yellow onion

1 large green chili (stem and seeds removed and discarded), chopped

1/4 c. water

1/4 c. cilantro, chopped

Pinch of cayenne pepper

Salt to taste

In a large frying pan, sauté olive oil and onions to lightly browned. Then add the garlic, tomatoes, chayotes, green chili, water, and cayenne. Simmer for 10 minutes, stirring occasionally to avoid burning. Remove from heat and serve with cilantro.

Servings: 4

Chayote

Chayotes, also known as "vegetable pears," are related to zucchini, cucumber, and melons, and in a way, taste like a combination of all three. They are a staple of Mexico and Costa Rica, are high in vitamin C, low in calories, and are a good source of fiber. They can be eaten raw, or cooked, and like zucchini, baked, broiled, sautéed, steamed, or mashed. The skins can be tough (they grow well in intense sunlight and hot environments); best when peeled.

Pico de Gallo

6 plum (Roma) tomatoes, diced
1/2 red onion, minced
3 Tbsps. fresh cilantro, chopped
1/2 jalapeno pepper, seeded and minced
1/2 lime, juiced
2 cloves garlic, minced
1 pinch ground cumin
Salt and ground black pepper to taste

In a mixing bowl, stir the tomatoes, onion, cilantro, jalapeno pepper, lime juice, garlic, cumin, salt, and pepper together.

Refrigerate at least 3 hours before serving to allow the flavors to mingle.

Use as a dip or a side-sauce for eggs, beans, or other foods.

Servings: 10-12

Cilantro

This herb and the seeds from it (coriander) have powerful anti-inflammatory capacities that help relieve symptoms of arthritis, increase HDL cholesterol (the good kind), and reduces LDL cholesterol (the bad kind), and helps reduce feelings of nausea. Cilantro is an excellent source of iron and magnesium. It will relieve diarrhea, helps promote healthy liver function, and disinfects and helps detoxify the body. In addition, it contains immune-boosting properties.

Quinoa with Tahini Garlic Sauce

2-1/4 c. vegetable broth or water
1-1/2 c. quinoa
1 bunch fresh spinach, coarsely chopped
1/3 c. tahini
1-2 cloves garlic, minced
2 Tbsps. fresh lemon juice
1/4 tsp. sea salt, or to taste

Boil the vegetable broth or water, then add quinoa and reduce the heat to a simmer and cover for 10-15 minutes. Turn off the heat and keep covered for 5 more minutes. Add the spinach to the steaming quinoa and cover for 4 minutes.

Place tahini in a small bowl. Stir in minced garlic, lemon juice and salt. Gradually stir in 2-3 tablespoons (or more if necessary) hot water until it becomes a creamy sauce. Serve the quinoa and spinach topped with tahini sauce.

Servings: 4

Source: vegancoach.com

Quinoa

Although referred to as a grain, quinoa is actually a seed from a vegetable related to Swiss chard, spinach and beets. It is a high quality protein with nine essential amino acids, a protein balance similar to milk. Quinoa is a great source of riboflavin and is alkaline-forming, at least comparable to wild rice, amaranth, and sprouted grains. Since it is not related to wheat, or even a grain, it is gluten-free.

Rice Noodles with Walnut Pesto

3 c. packed fresh basil leaves
3 large cloves garlic
1/3 c. walnuts
1/3 c. extra virgin olive oil
1/3 c. grated parmesan cheese
Additional extra-virgin olive oil (for storage)
8 oz. rice noodles
Salt and pepper to taste

Walnut pesto: Place the basil leaves and garlic in a food processor or blender, and mix well.

Add the walnuts, and continue to blend until the walnuts are finely ground. Keep the machine running as you drizzle in the olive oil. When you have a smooth paste, transfer to a bowl, and stir in the parmesan cheese. Season to taste with salt and pepper.

If all the pesto is not used for this dish, dribble additional oil to cover and seal, then refrigerate in a covered container and serve with other dishes, especially eggs or brown rice.

Rice noodles: Place noodles in a pot or bowl of hot water 5-12 minutes, or just until noodles are soft enough to eat, but still firm and a little bit chewy. Drain and briefly rinse noodles with cold water to stop the cooking.

In a bowl, spoon in a generous portion of the pesto. Add noodles and gently mix. Use more pesto to taste.

Servings: 2-3

Sesame Broccoli

1 c. water
1 lb. fresh broccoli spears
1 Tbsp. sesame seeds
4 tsps. extra virgin olive oil, divided
1 Tbsp. lemon juice

In a large saucepan, bring water to a boil. Add broccoli. Reduce heat. Cover and simmer for 5-7 minutes or until crisp-tender.

While the broccoli is cooking, in a small skillet, sauté sesame seeds in 1 teaspoon of the oil until lightly browned. Remove from the heat. Stir in the lemon juice and remaining oil. Drain broccoli, then toss with sesame seed mixture.

Servings: 4-5

Sesame seeds

Sesame seeds contain sesame-lignin, which helps the body eliminate the free radicals that cause aging and cancer, including fatty acid production. Sesame seeds also contain phytate, one of the most powerful antioxidants and one of the most potent natural anti-cancer substances, which helps inhibit the growth of various cancer cells. Overall, sesame seeds provide optimum vitality and strength. For chemo patients, they help to relieve constipation, softening the stool.

Sautéed Kale

2-3 Tbsps. olive oil
2-3 cloves of garlic, minced
1 head kale, deveined, chopped
Sea salt to taste

In a large frying pan, sauté garlic for about 30 seconds. Add the kale and cook until tender. Salt and serve.

Servings: 4-6

Source: Jen Klien – sheknows.com

Kale. *Called "the queen of greens," kale is a nutritional powerhouse. One cup of kale has only 36 calories and 0 grams of fat, but an impressive 5 grams of fiber. It is great for aiding in digestion and elimination with its great fiber content. Kale is high in iron (per calorie, more than beef). Kale is filled with powerful antioxidants, such as carotenoids and flavonoids that help protect against various cancers. It is a great anti-inflammatory food. Kale is high in vitamin C, which helps supports the immune system and aids in hydration.*

Biryani Rice

1-1/2 c. brown rice, cooked with cinnamon stick

1/2 c. peas

1 onion, finely chopped

2 tomatoes, finely chopped

2 garlic cloves, minced

1 tsp. ginger root, minced

1 cinnamon stick

1 bay leaf

6-8 black peppercorns

4 cloves

1/2 tsp. cumin seeds

1 Tbsp. coriander powder

1/2 tsp. paprika

1/4 tsp. turmeric

1/2 c. cilantro chopped

2 Tbsps. coconut oil

4 c. water

Heat coconut oil in a frying pan. Add the bay leaf, cumin seeds, black peppercorns, cloves and chopped onions and sauté them till onions are browned. Add ginger and garlic along with turmeric powder, paprika, coriander powder and sauté for 3-4 minutes. Finally, add the chopped tomatoes and salt. Cook on medium heat covered until the tomatoes are soft and broken down and the oil starts to show on the surface, about 10 minutes. Now add the peas and cook for another minute or so. Make sure to keep stirring to avoid the mixture from burning. Once the tomato mixture is well done, add the cooked rice and chopped cilantro, mix. Serve hot. Servings: 4

Source: Reem Rizvi – simplyreem.com, adapted by Dr. Mike

Turmeric

Turmeric is a potent natural antiseptic and antibacterial agent, useful topically in disinfecting cuts and burns. Turmeric may prevent melanoma and cause existing melanoma cells to commit suicide. It is a natural liver detoxifier. New research is showing that it may prevent metastases from occurring in many different forms of cancer. Turmeric boosts the effects of the chemo drug paclitaxel and reduces its side effects.

Roasted Brussels Sprouts with Fennel and Shiitake Mushrooms

1-1/2 lbs. Brussels sprouts
4 shallots, quartered
10 garlic cloves, peeled
1/2 pound shiitake mushroom caps
1 large fennel bulb
1/4 c. extra virgin olive oil
3 Tbsps. balsamic vinegar
2 Tbsps. fresh tarragon or rosemary
Salt and pepper to taste

Preheat oven to 425 degrees. Prepare Brussels sprouts by cutting away tough root ends and removing any blemished outer leaves. Slice in half through the base and place in large bowl. Add shallots, garlic and mushroom caps. Prepare fennel by trimming off dried root end and slicing bulb thinly width-wise. Add to vegetables and toss with olive oil, vinegar, tarragon, and salt and pepper to taste. Place in 9 x 12 inch glass or ceramic baking dish and roast uncovered 25 minutes. Stir vegetables and roast 25 minutes more. Remove from oven and serve.

Servings: 6

Source: Terry Walters – terrywalters.net

Sweet Potato Oven Baked Fries

1 sweet potato, cleaned, not peeled
2 Tbsps. olive oil or coconut oil
1 tsp. dried rosemary
1/2 tsp. sea salt

Preheat the oven to 400 degrees. Cut the sweet potatoes in to 1/4 inch strips that resemble traditional French fries. In a large bowl, add the oil, rosemary, and salt. Stir. Add potatoes and mix until the potatoes are evenly coated with oil and herbs. Place on a cookie sheet in a single layer. Bake for 15 minutes. Then flip the sweet potatoes over to brown the other side and place back in the oven for about 15 more minutes. Check them every 5 minutes to ensure they don't burn.

Servings: 2

Sea salt

Sea salt balances the body with minerals. In conjunction with water and in the right proportion, sea salt is essential for the regulation of blood pressure. It supplies essential minerals directly to the cells to enhance and improve the immune system and increases resistance against infections and bacterial diseases. It acts as a strong natural antihistamine by maintaining the body's acidic level and preventing different health problems and degenerative diseases.

Tasty Tabouli Salad

3/4 c. boiling water

1/2 c. bulgur wheat

1 c. parsley, minced

1/4 c. mint leaves, minced

1/2 c. spring onions, minced

1 tomato, diced

3 tsps. olive oil

1-2 Tbsps. lemon juice

1 tsp. sea salt

1 clove garlic, chopped finely

Pepper and paprika to taste

Pour boiling water over bulgur wheat, cover, and let stand about 20 minutes until wheat is tender and most of the water is absorbed. Add parsley, garlic, mint, onion, and tomato. Toss to mix. Combine olive oil, lemon juice, salt, and pepper/paprika. Add to wheat mixture. Chill in fridge until cool, then serve. For an extra crunch, try adding some diced cucumber at the end. It provides an extra fresh, cool burst of flavor for the Tabouli salad.

Servings: 3-4

Source: Dr. Tom Corson - tomcorsonknowles.com

Quinoa Tabouli

3 cloves garlic, minced
1 c. quinoa, cooked
1 cucumber, diced
2 tomatoes, diced
1/2 c. kalamata olives, diced
1/4 c. lemon juice
1 Tbsp. olive oil
Salt and pepper to taste

In a small skillet, add a few drops of olive oil. Warm over a low heat and add the garlic. Stir constantly until lightly browned. In a large bowl, add the lemon juice, olive oil, garlic, olives, cucumbers, and tomatoes. Mix in the quinoa. Stir and serve warm or cold.

Servings: 4

Source: Emily Molone – dailygarnish.com, adapted by Dr. Mike

Mushroom and Broccoli Salad

1 lb. broccoli, chopped course
4 oz. shiitake, stemmed and quartered
4 oz. enokitake, stems trimmed
1 c. green onions, thinly sliced
1/3 c. rice vinegar
2 tsp. minced fresh ginger
3/4 tsp. coarse salt
1/2 tsp. freshly ground pepper
3/4 c. extra virgin olive oil
2 tsp. sesame oil

Steam broccoli over simmering water until tender but still crisp, 3-4 minutes. Plunge into ice water to stop cooking and drain. In large bowl, combine broccoli, mushrooms, and green onions. In a medium bowl, mix vinegar with ginger, salt and pepper. Whisk in oils. Pour over vegetables and toss. Serve immediately.

Servings: 4

Source: adapted from **The Totally Mushroom Cookbook** *by Helene Siegel and Karen Gillingham (Berkeley, CA: Celestial Arts, 1994)*

Notes

Notes

SAUCES & DRESSINGS

Garden Fresh Salsa

2-3 medium tomatoes, finely chopped

1/2 c. onion, finely chopped

3 garlic cloves, minced

1 tsp. cider vinegar

1 tsp. lemon juice

1 Tbsp. extra virgin olive oil

1 tsp. jalapeno pepper, minced

1/2 tsp. salt

1/4 tsp. cayenne pepper

Mix all ingredients together in mixing bowl. Serve with rice crackers or baked corn tortillas.

Cayenne Pepper

Cayenne pepper is a miracle spice. It benefits the body's glandular, circulatory, lymphatic, and digestive systems. Cayenne is useful in alleviating allergies and muscle cramps, improving digestion, and helping wound healing. From helping to cure the common cold to fighting fatigue, cayenne is king.

Fast Red Sauce

10 medium tomatoes, coarsely chopped
1 red onion, finely chopped
4-5 garlic cloves, minced
4-5 fresh basil leaves, chopped
2 Tbsps. Italian seasoning
2 Tbsps. olive or coconut oil
1 tsp. oregano
Salt to taste

Place the tomatoes and seasonings in a blender. Blend on a medium speed for chunky consistency. Heat the oil in a large frying pan on medium heat. Add the onions and cook until translucent. Add the garlic and the blended tomatoes. Let simmer for 10 minutes. Add salt and fresh basil leaves. Serve warm. Great over steamed vegetables, spaghetti squash, brown rice, rice noodles, quinoa, or as a soup base.

Servings: 4-5

Arugula Pesto

1 c. fresh arugula
1/2 c. fresh cilantro
4 walnuts, chopped
1 garlic clove
1 Tbsp. lemon juice
4 Tbsps. extra-virgin olive oil
1/4 c. grated parmesan cheese
Pinch of sea salt

Place all ingredients in a food processer or blender. Mix until smooth.

Arugula pesto spices up any dish. Serve with brown rice or mixed with rice noodles.

Makes: 1 cup

Source: Kankana Saxena adapted by Dr. Mike

Extra Virgin Olive Oil

Extra virgin olive oil is different from all other oils (even other grades of olive oil) in that it is richly endowed with a unique combination of mono-unsaturated fats, polyphenols, and phytosterols. A huge volume of scientific studies shows that diets rich in these three natural components are associated with lower levels of "bad cholesterol" (LDL) and higher levels of "good cholesterol" (HDL)—and reduced DNA oxidative damage, which in turn is related to a reduced risk of some cancers.

Fresh Herbal Vinaigrette

1 garlic clove, minced
1 1/2 tsp. Dijon mustard
1 tsp. fresh thyme, minced
1 tsp. fresh oregano, minced
1 tsp. fresh basil, minced
1 tsp. fresh mint, minced
1 1/2 tsp. lemon juice
3 tsps. red wine vinegar
3/4 c. extra-virgin olive oil
Salt and pepper to taste

In a medium bowl, stir the garlic and Dijon mustard with a fork, creating a paste. Add the fresh herbs, lemon juice, and red wine vinegar. Stir. Whisk in the olive oil. Season with salt and pepper.

Fresh herbal vinaigrette keeps refrigerated for up to 1 week.

Makes: 1 cup

Source: Jessica Strand, from her book Salad Dressings *(San Francisco: Chronicle Books, 2007)*

Avocado Vinaigrette

2 garlic cloves

1 tsp. Dijon mustard

1 1/2 tsp. balsamic vinegar

2 1/2 tsp. lemon juice

Dash, Worcestershire sauce

1 avocado, peeled, pitted, and sliced into quarters

Pinch, cayenne pepper

3/4 c. virgin olive oil

1 tsp. lemon zest

Salt and pepper to taste

Put all the ingredients except the olive oil, zest, and black pepper into a blender or a food processor. Blend. Add the olive oil in a steady stream until the dressing emulsifies. Transfer into a medium bowl. Fold the zest in with a large spoon. Season with pepper.

Avocado Vinaigrette keeps refrigerated for 2-3 days.

Makes: 1 cup

Source: Jessica Strand, from her book **Salad Dressings** *(San Francisco: Chronicle Books, 2007)*

Garlic

Garlic has a distinguished body of scientific evidence promoting its general anti-cancer benefits, and there are good research reasons for classifying garlic as an anti-cancer food. A legendary immune-booster, garlic also has the ability to help treat bacterial infections that are difficult to heal because of the presence of bacteria that have become resistant to prescription antibiotics.

Roasted Red Pepper Vinaigrette

1 red bell pepper
2 garlic cloves
2 tsps. balsamic vinegar
1 tsp. fresh lemon juice
Tabasco sauce, dash
3/4 c. extra virgin olive oil
Salt and pepper to taste

Put the bell pepper on a fork and place it over a medium flame on the stove. When it blisters, turn it. Make sure all sides blister, and place it in a brown paper bag for 10 minutes. Cool. Remove the pepper from the bag, and peel, halve, and core. Put all the ingredients except the olive oil and black pepper into a blender or food processor. Blend. Add the olive oil in a steady stream until the dressing emulsifies. Transfer to a medium bowl. Season with pepper.

Roasted Red Pepper Vinaigrette keeps refrigerated for 2 weeks.

Makes: 1 cup

Source: Jessica Strand, from her book Salad Dressings *(San Francisco: Chronicle Books, 2007*

Sweet Red Peppers

A red pepper contains almost 300% of a body's required daily vitamin C intake. Besides being a powerful antioxidant, vitamin C is also needed for the proper absorption of iron. Red peppers are an excellent source of vitamin B6 and magnesium. Red peppers are one of the highest vegetable sources of lycopene, which has been successfully tested in the prevention of many cancers including prostate and lung.

Classic Caesar Dressing

3 garlic cloves

2 tsps. Dijon mustard

4 tsps. fresh lemon juice

2 egg yolks

Dash, Worcestershire sauce

6 anchovy fillets, chopped

1 Tbsp. freshly grated parmesan cheese

3/4 c. extra virgin olive oil

Salt and pepper to taste

Combine all the ingredients except the olive oil and black pepper in a blender or food processor. Mix. Add the olive oil in a steady stream until the dressing emulsifies. Transfer to a medium bowl. Season with pepper.

Classic Caesar Dressing keeps refrigerated for 5-7 days.

Makes: 1 cup

Eggs

One egg contains 6 grams of high-quality protein and all nine essential amino acids. One egg yolk has about 300 micrograms of choline, an important nutrient that helps regulate the brain, nervous system, and cardiovascular system. Eggs are one of the only foods that contain naturally occurring vitamin D. And eggs may prevent breast cancer—in one study, women who consumed at least six eggs per week lowered their risk of breast cancer by 44%.

Tahini Dressing

2 medium garlic cloves, minced

4 Tbsps. Tahini

6 Tbsps. olive oil

3 Tbsps. fresh lemon juice

2 Tbsps. fresh Italian parsley, minced

Salt and pepper to taste

In a medium bowl, combine all the ingredients and 3 tablespoons of water. To thin the sauce, add 1-2 tablespoons of water.

Tahini Dressing keeps refrigerated for 5-7 days.

Makes: 1 cup

Source: Jessica Strand, from her book Salad Dressings *(San Francisco: Chronicle Books, 2007), adapted by Dr. Mike*

Italian parsley

Parsley is a powerful immune-booster. Studies show that myristicin, an organic compound found in the essential oil of parsley, inhibits tumor formation. It is rich in antioxidants that include luteolin, a flavonoid that searches out and eradicates free radicals that cause oxidative stress in cells. In addition, parsley is an effective anti-inflammatory agent within the body. It is also an excellent source of valuable vitamin K.

Better-Than-Butter Garlic Spread

1 large garlic bulb
3/4 c. olive oil, cold pressed extra virgin
Sea salt

Pre-heat oven to 375 degrees. Place the whole garlic head on a cookie sheet. Bake for 8 minutes and turn off the oven. Let stand in the oven, 10-15 minutes. Remove the garlic and allow to cool. Peel or squeeze out the garlic pulp from the outer skins and/or blend in a blender with a high quality olive oil. Add salt. Blend on a slow to medium speed or mash by hand until smooth. Refrigerate in a glass jar. Use as a spread instead of butter.

Keeps refrigerated for up to 3 weeks.

Makes: 3/4 cup

Almondaise

1 ½ c. water
1/2 c. whole almond
1/2 tsp. salt
1 tsp. onion powder
1 tsp. mustard powder
1/2 c. olive oil
2 Tbsps. lemon juice

Bring 1 cup water and the almonds to a boil. Drain and rinse with cold water and remove skins. In blender or food processor, blend blanched almonds, 1/2 cup water, salt, onion powder and mustard powder. Blend until very smooth.

While blender is running, slowly pour in olive oil until mixture thickens. Pour into a bowl and fold in lemon juice.

Makes: 2 cups

Almonds

Almonds are an excellent source of vitamin E and manganese, magnesium, copper, riboflavin (vitamin B2), and phosphorus. Fortunately, although one-quarter cup of almonds contains about 18 grams of fat, most of it (11 grams) is heart-healthy monounsaturated fat. Almonds are concentrated in protein. A quarter-cup contains 7.62 grams—more protein than a typical egg, which contains 5.54 grams.

Notes

SNACKS

Brown Rice Cake Snacks

1. Brown rice cake with almondaise (see Sauces and Dressings), topped with fresh-grown sprouts.

2. Brown rice cake with almond cream and a few berries satisfies the afternoon sweet tooth. This is a light snack that can double as a nice dessert.

3. Brown rice cake with leftover beans (mashed) and arugula with garden fresh salsa makes a quick snack or a light lunch when served with steamed vegetables or large green salad.

4. My personal favorite is brown rice cake with almond butter and mashed berries. This old time child's favorite is very comforting.

Serves: 1

Brown Rice

Rice is one of nature's perfect foods. In about half the world, "to eat" means "to eat rice." Rich in fiber and selenium, brown rice is an important dietary source of water-soluble antioxidants. The antioxidants are both immediate-release and slow-release, and so are available throughout the gastrointestinal tract over a long period after eating.

Baked Crispy Kale

4 large handfuls of kale, torn into bite-sized pieces and tough stems removed (about 1/3 pound)
1-2 Tbsps. olive oil
Sea salt or kosher salt

Preheat oven to 350 degrees. Line a baking sheet with parchment paper. Place the kale leaves into a salad spinner and spin all of the water out of the kale. Repeat a few times to ensure there are no water traces on the leaves.

In a large bowl, drizzle olive oil over the kale leaves and hand toss to coat the leaves. Bake on the lined baking sheet in the oven for 12-20 minutes until leaves are crisp. Take a peek at the 12-minute mark. The timing all depends on how much olive oil is used. Just use a spatula or tongs to touch the leaves; if they are paper-thin crackly, the kale is done. If the leaves are still a bit soft, leave them in for another 2 minutes. Do not let the leaves turn brown (they'll be bitter.) Salt and cool before eating.

Serves: 4

Source: Jaden Hair – steamykitchen.com

Jicama Sticks with Lime Juice

1 jicama, peeled, cut into sticks
1 lime, juiced
Sea salt to taste

Prepare the jicama into sticks or bite-size cubes and place in a bowl. Juice the lime over the jicama. Mix to coat evenly. Then add the salt. Mix again.

Serves: 2

Jicama

A cup of jicama has only 46 calories, but this root has many health benefits, including providing an excellent source of fiber. Jicama contains generous amounts of vitamins C and E, potassium, and iron. With its high content of vitamin C, it is a great antioxidant and immune booster, helping the overall function of the body.

Nori Roll with Brown Rice, Avocado, and Cucumber

3 nori sheets
1 c. brown rice, cooked
1 avocado, pitted, peeled, sliced
1/2 cucumber, peeled, sliced thin
3 tsps. sesame seeds

Place one nori sheet on the counter and add a few teaspoons of rice in the middle of the sheet in a line. Stack the avocado and cucumber along the line of rice and sprinkle with sesame seeds. Bend the nori sheet over the rice line to form a tube. Then slide the top layer of the nori back to tighten the ingredients in the roll. (A sushi roller may be used.) Moisten the end of the nori sheet with a bit of water to seal the roll closed.

Makes: 3 rolls

Hummus

1-1/2 c. dried garbanzo beans
1/2 c. sesame seeds
1-2 large cloves garlic
1 c. water
1 tsp. cumin
1 tsp. fresh Italian parsley
Sprinkle of cayenne pepper
Salt

Fill a bowl with water and soak the dry garbanzo beans 24 hours or more in the refrigerator. After soaking, drain reserving ½ cup of water. Blend beans with the water.

Grind sesame seeds in a coffee or spice grinder to make a powder.

Mix all the ingredients, adding water to make a spreadable consistency. Add salt to taste.

Garnish with Italian parsley or cayenne pepper

Serve cold with baked corn chips or fresh cut carrots, celery, and jicama sticks.

Serves: 6

Rice Paper Wraps

Rice paper
1 avocado
1 cucumber
1 c. bean or alfalfa sprouts
1 medium tomato
Sprinkle of cayenne pepper

Slice avocado, cucumber and tomato into long, thin slices.

Soften rice paper according to directions on the package. Best is to run paper one piece at a time over warm water until pliable (but not so soggy that it breaks apart).

Add all ingredients to the center of the rice paper, fold the ends, and roll up. The paper should seal itself—if not, moisten a bit to seal.

Serve as a lunch with cold or hot soup, or as an afternoon snack.

Serves: 2

Health Snack Mix

1 c. shelled walnuts

1/2 c. almonds

1/2 c. dried cranberries

1/2 c. yellow raisins

1/2 c. unsalted, roasted pumpkin seeds

1 c. toasted oats

Pinch of sea salt to taste

Toast the oats by heating in a skillet, stirring constantly. Cool to room temperature.

In a large mixing bowl, mix all the ingredients together.

Serve as a snack throughout the day or as a topping for breakfast oatmeal.

Serves: 4

Notes

Notes

DESSERTS

Raw Chocolate Truffles

1 c. nut milk mash (pulp left from making Almond Milk)

1/2 c. raw Tahini

1/4 c. raw cacao powder (Raw cacao is ground from cacao beans. *The powder tastes similar to, but better than, unsweetened baker's chocolate.*)

1/4 c. raw agave to sweeten

2 Tbsps. coconut butter (optional)

Sea salt, pinch (optional)

1 tsp. vanilla extract

Almond milk (if needed)

Extra raw carob or cacao powder in a shallow dish.

Put first seven ingredients (counting the salt) in a bowl and mix together. Add a little nut milk if the consistency is too dry (you want the mix to be somewhat dry so you can roll it out easily). Roll into balls and then roll into cacao powder to cover. When your inner chocolate lover needs a kiss, this is a very special treat!

Servings: 10 or more

Source: Linda Wooliever - vt-fiddle.com

Basic Chocolate Cake

---

4 c. nut mash (2 c. almonds, 2 c. hazelnuts)
1/2-3/4 c. coconut oil
2 rounded Tbsps. cacao powder
1 tsp. vanilla extract
Sea salt, pinch

Place all ingredients in a bowl and mix with an electric mixer until smooth and creamy texture has formed. Add a small amount of nut milk if it looks too dry. The coconut oil will help to solidify it, however, if you want an even fudgier mixture, add 1/4-1/2 cup raw nut butter to the mix and hand-mix it together.

Spread the mixture evenly in the bottom of a springform pan. If the fudge is too sticky to spread, put your spatula or rubber scraper under some cold water and it will spread more easily with no sticking. Refrigerate before serving and store refrigerated.

Servings: 8-10

Source: Linda Wooliever - vt-fiddle.com

Chocolate Pudding

2 bananas

1 avocado

1-2 Tbsp. raw cacao powder (or raw carob)

1 tsp. raw honey or agave (optional)

Mix in a food processor until it becomes smooth, like pudding.

Servings: 2

Source: Linda Wooliever - vt-fiddle.com

Strawberry Tapioca

1 c. fresh strawberries
1 c. tapioca pearls
1 tsp. natural vanilla extract
Sprig of fresh mint

Soak strawberries in water, drain, trim stems from strawberries, slice into halves, and place in refrigerator.

To prepare the tapioca, use 1/2 cup tapioca pearls to 2 cups water (or follow directions on package). Soak pearls in water for 20 minutes, drain. Heat 2 cups water to boiling in a saucepan, add tapioca pearls. Cook for 10 minutes, stirring attentively. Stir in the vanilla.

While the tapioca is still warm, spoon into a parfait dish, top with the fresh strawberries. Add a sprig of mint for garnish.

Tapioca

One of the great benefits of tapioca is that is fills the need for a sweet tooth, but does so without the issues associated with sugar and sugar substitutes. As a dietary starch, it offers nutritional bonuses similar to other starchy root vegetables, such as potatoes. With fruit, it makes a delicious and filling dessert.

Barley Scones (contains gluten)

1/4 c. almond or rice milk

2 Tbsps. maple syrup

1 Tbsp. organic coconut oil

2 tsps. vinegar

1 c. plus 3 Tbsp. barley flour

1/4 tsp. baking soda

1 tsp. baking powder (aluminum free)

1/4 tsp. salt

3 Tbsps. raisins

Barley flour for dusting

Preheat oven to 350 degrees. Mix milk, maple syrup, oil, and vinegar. Set aside. Combine flour, baking soda, salt, and raisins in a food processor. Blend until well mixed and raisins are chopped. Add liquid ingredients and process until a ball of dough forms.

Transfer to a flat surface that has been dusted with barley flour. Flatten into a circle approximately 6 inches in diameter and 3/4-inch thick. Use a sharp knife to score dough into 12 wedges (do not separate), then transfer to a baking sheet. Bake for 30 minutes, until lightly browned.

Servings: 12 or more

Source: **Healthy Eating for Life for Women by the Physicians** *Committee for Responsible Medicine, Kris Kieswer, ed. (Hoboken, NJ: Wiley, 2002)*

Butternut Squash with Walnuts and Berries

4 c. water

1 butternut squash, peeled, seeds removed, chopped

1 heaping c. of walnuts, chopped

2 Tbsps. organic coconut oil

2-3 tsps. ginger, grated

1-2 tsps. pure vanilla extract

1/2 lemon or lime, juiced (optional)

1-2 tsps. cinnamon

1/2 c. fresh or frozen cranberries or blueberries

Salt to taste

In a large soup pot, add the water and chopped squash. Boil for 10 minutes, covered. Strain water; add berries, if frozen, and coconut oil. Cover to let steam for just a minute. (If fresh berries are being used add them at the very end.)

Mix ginger, walnuts, pure vanilla extract, cinnamon and lime or lemon juice together and add to the steamed squash mix. Add the fresh berries. Gently mix together.

Served warm or cold. Makes a great breakfast with granola and almond milk.

Servings: 4

Grilled Apples

1 red or green apple, sliced 1/4 inch thick
Cinnamon
Almond milk
Dried cranberries

Place on a gas grill, electric grill or grilling pan for three minutes per side or until the grill marks are present and the apple is slightly cooked.

Sprinkle with dried cranberries, drizzle with almond milk and dust with cinnamon.

Servings: 1-2

Dried cranberries

After extensive research, dried cranberries have been linked to health benefits such as strengthening the immune system, and battling against bacterial and viral infections. Dried cranberries contain abundant amounts of vitamin C and antioxidants. These help decrease the effect of free radicals in the body, which in turn limits the development of cancer cells.

Chocolate Strawberry Milkshake

1 c. almond, oat, or seed milk

1 c. ice cubes or frozen cubes of almond milk or seed milk

1 tsp. pure vanilla extract

1 tsp. cacao powder (optional)

5 fresh strawberries (optional)

Place all ingredients in the blender and blend until smooth. Adjust the thickness with more ice or almond/seed milk.

Serving: 1

Strawberries

Strawberries contain a wide range of nutrients, with vitamin C heading the list. They also contain significant levels of phytonutrients and antioxidants, which fight free radicals. In addition to vitamin C, strawberries also provide an excellent source of vitamin K and manganese, as well as folic acid, potassium, riboflavin, vitamin B5, vitamin B6, copper, magnesium, and omega 3 fatty acids.

Oatmeal Cookies

2 c. oatmeal, cooked

1 tsp. cinnamon

1 egg

1/2 tsp. aluminum-free baking soda

2 Tbsps. organic agave nectar

1/2 c. walnuts, chopped

1/4 c. raisins (optional)

Salt, pinch

Preheat the oven to 350 degrees. In a large mixing bowl, add all ingredients and mix together well. Grease a cookie sheet with coconut oil. Spoon out the cookie batter and place on the cookie sheet about 1 inch apart from each other. Bake for 8-12 minutes or until golden brown.

Makes: 20 cookies

Raisins

Raisins are concentrated sources of energy, vitamins, minerals, and antioxidants. They contain the phytochemical compound resveratrol, a polyphenol antioxidant that has anti-inflammatory, anti-cancer, blood cholesterol-lowering abilities. Studies suggest that resveratrol can protect against melanoma, and colon and prostate cancer. Raisins are dense sources of minerals like calcium, iron, manganese, magnesium copper and zinc.

Soft Almond Cookies

2 c. almond pulp (strained from making almond milk)
3 tsps. agave nectar
1 tsp. aluminum-free baking soda
3 Tbsps. almond butter
1 egg
1 tsp. pure vanilla extract
1 c. toasted amaranth
Salt, pinch

Preheat the oven to 350 degrees. Toast the amaranth in a medium size frying pan on a medium heat, stirring constantly, until the amaranth turns slightly golden color and makes a popping sound. In a large mixing bowl, add all ingredients and mix together well.

Oil a cookie sheet with coconut oil. Spoon out the cookie batter and place on the cookie sheet about 1 inch apart from each other. Bake in the oven for 18-23 minutes or until golden brown.

Remove from cookie sheet and place on cooling rack.

Makes: 20 cookies.

Mint Chocolate Chip Shake

1 Tbsp. raw cacao nibs

1/2 tsp. vanilla extract

1 c. or more unsweetened almond milk

1 handful mint leaves (stems OK too)

2 tsps. green food supplement (optional)

5 large ice cubes

Pinch of sea salt

Combine all ingredients in a blender, and blend until smooth. Thin out with more almond milk if needed.

Serving: 1

Source: Adapted from Cafe Gratitude – cafegratitude.com

Chia Pudding

2/3 c. chia seeds

2 c. unsweetened non-dairy milk (almond, rice, or oat milk)

1/2 tsp. pure vanilla extract

2 Tbsps. currants or chopped dried figs or dates

2 Tbsps. unsweetened coconut flakes

Place chia seeds, almond milk and vanilla in a 1-quart glass jar with a lid. Tighten the lid and shake well to thoroughly combine.

Or, stir together seeds, almond milk, and vanilla in a bowl and refrigerate overnight. When ready to serve, stir well. Spoon into bowls and top with fruit and coconut.

Servings: 6

Source: Whole Foods - wholefoodsmarket.com

Chia Seed Delight

1/4 c. raw, organic chia seeds
1 c. almond milk
1/3 Tbsp. raw cacao powder
Stevia or xylitol to sweeten

Place chia seeds in a bowl. Blend the almond milk, cacao powder and stevia or xylitol in the blender until mixed well and desired level of sweetness is reached. Pour over chia seeds and mix well. Let stand for at least 15 minutes before mixing again and serving.

Serving: 1

Source: Kimberly Snyder - kimberlysnyder.net

Chia

Chia seeds are loaded with antioxidants, vitamins, minerals, and fiber. They feature a perfect balance of essential fatty acids: 30% of chia seed oil is omega 3 oil and 40% is omega 6 oil. Studies also show that eating chia seed slows down our bodies' conversion of carbohydrate calories into simple sugars. This is great for preventing spikes in blood sugar, whether you are diabetic or not.

PART FOUR

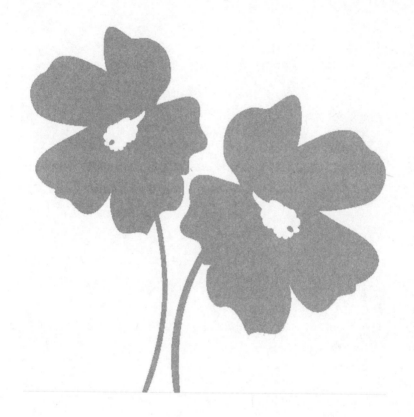

Beyond Chemotherapy

PART FOUR

Beyond Chemotherapy

Live in rooms full of light

Avoid heavy food

Be moderate in the drinking of wine

Take massage, baths, exercise, and gymnastics

Fight insomnia with gentle rocking or the sound of running water

Change surroundings and take long journeys

Strictly avoid frightening ideas

Indulge in cheerful conversation and amusements

Listen to music

A. Cornelius Celsus

The Future

In a personal war against cancer, the first casualty is the future.

For someone diagnosed with cancer, time seems to stop and life is put on hold. Instead of dreaming about next month, next year, or the next ten years, the stream of time stops abruptly as the mind comes ever back to today, tomorrow, the next day. What might have been imagined for life's goals and accomplishments suddenly boils down to meeting doctor's appointments, picking up prescriptions, showing up for blood work, getting scans.

The first order of business for the newly identified "cancer survivor," then, is to recover the future.

In this final section of the book, I am going to address the near future, the process of going from a cancer patient to cancer survivor, with emphasis on living a high quality life after chemotherapy. Then I will have some things to say about the future in general.

Change Your Identity

"People generally seem to adjust to the fact that they have cancer, but they don't adjust well to a life marked by disability. Why not?" asks Julie Silver, MD, author of *You Can Heal Yourself: A Guide to Physical and Emotional Recovery After Injury or Illness*. "Perhaps it is because cancer is virtually the only diagnosis in which patients are told to go home and figure out on their own how to heal. It has long been the practice to send cancer patients home after treatments—when they are sicker than they have ever been—and to tell them to 'accept a new normal.'"

There is a huge gap in conventional cancer treatment, and that is what happens after an oncologist judges a patient to be "cancer free," or at least to be showing no signs of cancer. In virtually every case, the picture is how Dr. Silver paints it: except for directions about getting regular check-ups at one-month, three-month, or six-month intervals, little guidance is given about how to live after cancer. Some of the major medical institutions have begun to address this issue, but much more still needs to be done.

The essential first step for a cancer patient becoming a cancer survivor is to consciously take on the new identity and to own it.

That means altering the way we identify ourselves in our speech—to ourselves and others. Once it was, "I have cancer"; now it is, "I had cancer." It sounds easy to do, but for someone slowly leaving the cloud of cancer treatment, it can take some time to process.

One thing to consider doing at this transitional point is to change your wardrobe, or at least some important parts of it. Getting new clothes always signifies a new identity. We are told by dream analysts that when we dream about putting on a new set of clothes, it means that we have begun to forge a new persona for ourselves.

In the gangster movies of the 1930s, an obligatory scene had the small-time hooligan being initiated into the large crime organization; the boss peels off a few big bills, tosses them at the lout and tells him to get an expensive suit, shirt, and tie. It pointed to a ritual that is everywhere in life, from the new recruit putting on a military uniform to the Catholic cardinal who has been elected Pope doffing his red vestments and putting on the white robes of his new office.

I advise my clients who have gone through chemotherapy and have come out of it healed of cancer to pack away (or throw away) the clothes they wore during treatment and dress in some new clothes. Doing this mindfully can be a powerful symbol that you are ready to leave the past behind and enter a bright new chapter of life.

When we entered the world of chemotherapy, we were startled, even shocked, to see the person—bald and often pasty and bloated from the drugs—staring back at us in the mirror. Now, as our body begins to be recognizable again, the deceptively simple act of dressing differently so that we appear changed in the mirror jump-starts us into forming new attitudes and beliefs about ourselves. The new person, dressed differently and beginning to look more "normal," is a glimpse into the future.

Make Your "Story" a Short Story

There are more than 12 million cancer survivors in the United States—and more than 12 million stories about being diagnosed, undergoing treatment, and coming out the other end "cancer free."

Most people like to talk about their illness, particularly when it is in the past tense. Visiting with friends and family during and after a cancer crisis, telling our "story" is inevitable. We tell it so often, sometimes with embellishments, sometimes glossing over facts, that it becomes as familiar as a memorized script.

I encourage my clients who have come through cancer to consider telling their story as a short story—not a long one. The reason is that every time we tell our story, it gets ingrained in us as part of who we are. Repeating it over and over, often with ever-increasing drama, tends to crowd out everything else about us. We become "professional cancer victims," with a one-note song. Try putting the recent past behind you while you are telling the same painful cancer story again and again. It's hard to do—maybe impossible.

I do not mean to imply that telling the story of your recovery is not important, to you and to others. A story with a happy ending is always a victory for everyone who hears it. In fact, speaking about your experiences or blogging about them on the Internet can give emotional support to others.

But I caution my cancer-survivor clients about becoming too attached to their story on the grounds that it might box them into a definition of themselves that can limit the way they regard the future. At this point, post-chemo and post-cancer, you are turning your attention away from disease and toward a positive future of well-being.

Get Moving

"It's really important to be obsessive about what [cancer survivors] do for themselves," says Nagi Kumar, a Professor in Oncologic Sciences at the University of South Florida. "Give it your all: do yoga, get more flexible, walk, eat right. Become very obsessive about what you're putting in your body."

"Physical activity is the clearest step you can take to benefit your health," writes Karen Syrjala, co-director of the Fred Hutchinson Cancer Research Center Survivorship Program. "It is certain to make you feel better and help your body and brain to function better. It can even reduce your cancer-related risks."

Exercise is tremendously beneficial for the continued well-being of cancer survivors. *The New York Times* reports a new study showing that exercise makes it less likely that a cancer survivor would later die from a recurrence of cancer. The lead author of the study was Dr. Rachel Ballard-Barbash, the associate director for applied research at the National Cancer Institute.

"When Dr. Ballard-Barbash and her colleagues teased out specific information about biomarkers related to cancer recurrence, they found that exercise tended reliably to improve insulin levels, reduce inflammation and increase populations of the very immune system cells that are thought to attack tumors," according to the *Times* report.

If you have been thinking that getting moving would wear you out, the exact opposite seems to be true. Another new study in Amsterdam has discovered that "exercise energizes people who are undergoing or have completed cancer treatment."

Getting physically on the move again after cancer also has symbolic steam behind it. Moving announces that the former cancer patient has returned to the world of the living, and is ready to begin being "a normal person" again.

Resume Life—Without Trying to Play "Catch-Up"

Once back in the swing of things, it is a good idea re-enter the stream of daily life, with all its various activities both exhilarating and mundane, gradually and at a comfortable pace. Remember that a cancer survivor has not only survived cancer, but has survived cancer treatment, as well. The rigors of chemotherapy and other cancer therapies are intense; they take a huge toll on the body, mind, and spirit.

"While I was having chemo, I quit doing almost everything. So when treatment ended, the challenge for me was, what am I going to do now with my life? What should I go back to doing?" This is a question asked by "Len," a cancer survivor on the website of the National Cancer Institute. It is a question that invariably comes to mind with all survivors: how do I pick up my life and at what point?

One of the hardest things after treatment is not knowing what happens next, the National Cancer Institute goes on to say. "Because the doctors and nurses never told me what to expect, I had very unrealistic expectations of wellness, and so did my family and friends," says another survivor. "This led to a great deal of worry."

When we receive a diagnosis of cancer, it is as if we place a bookmark in the life we were leading. At the end of the cancer experience, whether it lasted six months or a year, or several years, we expect that we can pick up our life at the place where we bookmarked it. But time has gone by. Family and friends and work associates have gone on with their lives—and their own triumphs and tragedies.

Rather than trying to play catch-up, it might be better to simply go easily with the flow, get back into things bit by bit, as stamina allows, and not worry about the time that seems to have been missed. The past is an illusion—no one lives there anymore. Re-entering the stream of life from where you are right now is the best way to sidestep feelings of exclusion.

Avoid "Drama"

Ask cancer survivors what they can tolerate the least after having coming through the dreaded disease and its often grueling treatment, and most will tell you, "drama." Cancer carries its own dramatic impact on our lives. When treatment is over, good health is returning, and we are settling down to a peaceful new life, the last thing we want around is someone who overreacts to or greatly exaggerates the importance of non-threatening events.

Psychologists tell us that "drama" is used by people who are chronically bored or who seek attention by trying to make their own lives seem more exciting. They have a whole catalog of "serious" problems, whether real or imaginary, and they dump them on others at the least provocation.

I counsel survivor clients to simply let drama-prone friends or family members quietly leave their lives. This can be done politely, by pleading fatigue or some other side effect of treatment. If that does not work, there are always firmer ways to protect oneself from a potentially upsetting person or situation. Saying "no" to an invitation to go out or to a home-visit from a drama queen or king is always permissible for a cancer survivor.

Some advice from the online Urban Dictionary: hold your trusted friends close to you, keep secrets, avoid arguments, don't lie, and, probably most important, stay out of other people's dramas.

The stress brought on by drama—trying to win an argument that is basically meaningless, for instance—will cause damage to the body. For one thing, under such stress nutrients from food and supplements do not get absorbed properly, leaving the immune system compromised.

Unnecessary emotional turmoil is exactly what a cancer survivor does not need. There has been quite enough of that already through the fearful days and months of the disease and the rigors of its treatment—enough to last a lifetime.

Look to the Future

Back to the future. One of the most beneficial exercises a cancer survivor can engage in is dreaming about the future. And not only dreaming about it, but taking it out of the realm of the imagination and putting it down on paper. Making plans is an essential element in healing.

"Losing hope is a dear price to pay," says Aaron in *Psychology Today*. "Ideals provide hope and a reference point for a better situation. The loss of hope, which is the loss of the capacity to imagine that things can be better, is a most profound type of loss—perhaps the most tragic kind."

The ancients considered hope to be an indispensable psychological quality. In Greek mythology, Prometheus stole fire from the gods. To punish him for his infraction, Zeus, king of the gods, created a box that contained all the evils that the gods had spared humankind. The box was entrusted to a young maiden, Pandora. She opened the box after being warned not to, and the evils were released into the world. By the time she was able to shut the box, only one item remained—and that was hope.

Two recent studies from the University of Queensland, the University of New South Wales, the Australian National University, and Monash University, have found that optimistic expectations are the key to making people happy with their lot in life. Professor Paul Frijters, one of the authors of the two studies, said a sample of over 10,000 Australians over nine years showed that people seemed to be better off if they expected good things to come.

Charles Snyder, one of the first developers of positive psychology, created his "hope theory," in which he described having goals as one of the greatest of human values. Based on many years of observation, Snyder made some suggestions about goals that can serve cancer survivors well. Among them:

- Recalling past successes—in this case, remembering good medical reports and feeling good on the "good days"

- Hearing stories of how other people have succeeded—from survivor friends or from movies, tapes, or books

- Exercising physically, relearning that the body and mind are connected

- Eating properly—rewarding the body with nutritious food for optimum functioning

- Resting adequately—sometimes easy to forget for someone who has come through cancer treatment and is feeling better and more energetic each day

- Laughing at oneself—the obligatory sense of humor, especially when we come up against limitations, finding that some goals will take longer to achieve than we had planned.

The best advice I can give to people who have been diagnosed with cancer, have gone through treatment, and come out of that experience returned to good health is—make plans for the future. Write them down, tell friends about them, research the Internet to see how you can implement them, imagine them actually unfolding in your life. You will see how this simple exercise can support your healing and bring you to that new level where you truly have left the past behind you.

And ancient proverb: He who has health has hope, and he who has hope has everything.

Create a Strategy for Life-Long Wellness

Finally, the way to go confidently into the bright future that lies ahead is to create a real plan for life-long wellness. That means, in most cases, that we cannot simply return to the lifestyle we lived before diagnosis and expect that we will live happily ever after. If we are to believe the rather convincing statistics, our pre-cancer lifestyle contributed greatly to the problem in the first place.

For a cancer survivor, living in optimum wellness calls for a strategy based on reliable knowledge and fired with an enthusiasm for having the best possible quality of life. This first post-cancer period should be taken up in great part with laying down the guidelines for staying well, enjoying high energy, relishing activity, and in general taking pleasure in life.

Naturally, regular medical check-ups are part of this scenario. If the doctor at the head of your healing team does not tell you exactly what do to upon leaving treatment, what dietary changes to make, when to report back, and so on, ask. This is important information for you and your caregiver. Be sure to have precise instructions regarding future blood work, scans, and doctor visits before walking out of the oncologist's office.

Here is my check-list for someone who has just received a "cancer free" ruling:

1. Create and maintain a physical activity that stimulates circulation, breathing, and chi (the energy centers in the body) such as

brisk walks, yoga, Pilates, swimming, and resistance training. Being physically active each day on a regular basis will help remove the toxic residue of the chemotherapy drugs and reduce the side effects of treatment.

2. Stay hydrated. The more purified water you drink, the quicker your body's cells will flush out any impurities that have accumulated before and during chemo rounds. Two to three liters of water per day will help detox your cells to allow for their optimal function.

3. Refrain from sugar of all forms. This includes artificial sweeteners as well as natural forms of sugar, such as white sugar, brown sugar, maple syrup, corn sugar, fructose, high fructose corn syrup, lactose (milk sugar), and high glycemic fruits and other foods. This will help "starve" cancer cells, limiting the likelihood of recurrence.

4. Stay on a limited animal protein diet, or discontinue animal proteins altogether (unless you have been a long-term vegan or vegetarian). Enjoy proteins from seeds, beans, nuts, and spirulina instead.

5. Eat a diet that contains 50% vegetables. Organic is best. All vegetable and fruits need to be cleaned before ingesting or preparing for cooking to avoid taking in any harmful bacteria.

6. Do not eat processed food, any food that is marketed to kids, or has unnatural colors. Artificial colors, preservatives, and additives cause cancer in small animals—and they have cells just as we do.

7. Eat homemade "real" foods. Most restaurants buy the cheapest ingredients and prepared sauces in huge factories miles away,

sauces that contain unhealthy ingredients that are created for flavor to keep their customers happy, not healthy.

8. Reduce your sodium intake. Normal table salt is enhanced with iodine. Iodine deficiency is less common now, but iodized salt is not as healthy as other options. Better choices are sea salt, rock salt, pink salt, or black salt, as they contain higher level of minerals.

9. Do coffee enemas. Even though your oncologist has given you great results, your liver (the largest filtration organ in the body) is still working overtime to cleanse your blood as a result of the chemotherapy doing its work. Dead cells get filtered through the liver. I suggest one enema per week for two months, and then once every two weeks for two months, followed by once a month as maintenance.

10. Supplements—specifically the supplements I recommend as part of this program—should be taken for at least two months beyond the last chemo day. They can be continued depending on the persistence of side effects. Brain fog, low energy, memory lapses, and the like will indicate that the supplements should be continued.

Finally, try to incorporate more joy time into your life. Laugh and smile at the little sparkles of unique opportunities for fun that are offered each day. People who look for joy will find it.

Start by loosening up and not taking life so seriously. Make funny faces in the mirror as a way to begin cultivating a joyful attitude. Dedicate yourself to activities you enjoy doing. All the research on this topic points in the same direction: happy people are less likely to be sick because joy elevates the immune system.

In a recent study, researchers at the University of Kentucky found that as subjects became more optimistic, they showed higher immunity to foreign viruses and bacteria. And when the subjects were not feeling so optimistic, their immunity dropped.

And there is data from Tel-Aviv University to support the hypothesis that individuals "characterized by a more negative affective style poorly recruit their immune response and may be at risk for illness more so than those with a positive affective style."

So, stay in joy. As the Greek poet, Pindar, wrote, "The best of healers is good cheer."

Acknowledgments, About the Authors, Bibliography

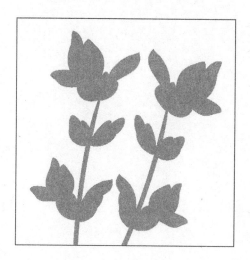

Acknowledgments

I would like to thank my parents, Sharron and Bill Herbert, for their love and support over the years, and particularly for opening their home as a place of healing during our cancer crisis. Truly, they helped to make this book possible in a fundamental way.

And Lorenzo Sandoval, a blind body worker and my first teacher, who encouraged me to pursue healing as a profession and service as a way of life.

Shari Reynolds, for the beautiful and intelligent design of this book and our website. And Lander Rodriguez for the book's interior design and Oscar Montes for photography and editorial support. And Stephanie Dagg, our Editorial Assistant

Also, the gifted naturopath Dana Kraft, nutritionist Kaayla Daniel for valuable advice, and these friends and champions: Andrea Usher, Ben Pitre, Helga and Bill Puschak, Jesse V. Castillo, Lynn Carlton, Laurel de Leo, Maria Belén Zavala Echeverria, Wade Ashley, and Dr. Scott Ulmer and his staff at the START Center for Cancer Care in San Antonio, Glenda Robinson, Dr. Beverly Nelson, Dr. Jeff Baldridge, Berenice Parra Vázquez, Stacy DeClercq, Ed and Cindy Carroll, the staff at Dos Casas in San Miguel de Allende, Dawn Gaskill, Dr. Ricardo Gordillo, Burton Goldberg, Elwood Richards, and K.C. Compton.

Special thanks to these professionals, who generously contributed recipes to the book: American Institute for Cancer Research, Cafe Gratitude (cafegratitude.com), chooseveg.com, Dr. Tom Corson (tomcorsonknowles.com), Emily Malone (dailygarnish.com), food.com, Jaden Hair (steamykitchen.com), Jen Klien (sheknows.com), Jennifer Raymond, M.S., R.D (cancerproject.org), Jessica Strand (Salad Dressings), Joe Cross and Phil Staples of the Reboot Your

Life Program, Kankana Saxena, Kimberly Snyder (kimberlysny-der.net), Kris Kieswer (*Healthy Eating for Life for Women*), Laurel De Leo, Linda Wooliever (vt-fiddle.com), Patty "Sassy" Knutson (vegancoach.com), Reem Rizvi (simplyreem.com), Terry Walters (terrywalters.net), Helene Siegel and Karen Gillingham (*The Total-ly Mushroom Cookbook*), Vegan Dinner Recipes (vegkitchen.com), Whole Foods (wholefoodsmarket.com).

Finally, I would like to acknowledge all the brave cancer patients and their caregivers who have to deal with not only the illness, but the huge amount of often conflicting, incomplete, and contradic-tory information on how to stay healthy during treatment. I wish you well on your journey to perfect and lasting well-being.

About the Authors

Mike Herbert is a Naturopathic Doctor and Certified Body Worker with fifteen years of experience in treating clients. He maintains a private practice in holistic wellness counseling.

Mike is dedicated to exploring the latest research in the fields of nutrition and natural healing. When his life was touched by a cancer crisis, he turned his full attention to investigating cutting-edge studies on the link between cancer and nutrition.

As a holistic practitioner, Mike believes that the true path of healing must include, along with the physical, the mental, emotional, and spiritual aspects of well-being. His many interests include physical conditioning, cooking, traveling, and experiencing different cultures.

Mike's degrees include a Bachelor of Science in Natural Health and a Doctorate of Naturopathy.

To learn more about Dr. Mike Herbert and his work, check out the website: stayhealthyduringchemo.com.

Before succumbing to cancer after years in remission, **Joseph Dispenza** (1942 – 2015) published several books and scores of articles about living a higher quality of life.

He was a former university film professor and former director of Education Programs for the American Film Institute.

Before moving to Santa Fe to write in the mid-1970s, he worked as a story editor for United Artists. In 2000, Joseph co-founded Life-Path Retreats in San Miguel de Allende and for about a decade conducted retreats based on The Way of the Traveler and Joseph Campbell's Hero's Journey.

Joseph was a columnist for several online publications, including Beliefnet. His articles appeared in magazines, including *Spirituality and Health*, *American Way*, *Massage Magazine*, and *Yoga Journal*. He also practiced independently as a spiritual counselor.

Bibliography

Abel, Emily K.; Subramanian, Saskia K. *After the Cure*. New York, NY: NYU Press, 2008

Alaoui-Jamali, Moulay A. *Alternative and Complementary Therapies for Cancer*. New York, NY: Springer, 2010.

Bagchi, Debasis; Preuss Harry G. *Phytopharmaceuticals in Cancer Chemoprevention*. Boca Raton, FL: CRC Press, 2004.

Barasi Mary E. *Human Nutrition*. London: Hodder Education, 2003.

Bendich, Adrianne; Deckelbaum, Richard J. *Preventive Nutrition*. New York, NY: Springer, 2005.

Berkson, Burt. *The Alpha Lipoic Acid Breakthrough*. New York, NY: Crown Publishing Group, 2010.

Betty Crocker Editors. *AARP Living with Cancer Cookbook*. New York: John Wiley & Sons, LTD., 2011.

Beuth, Josef; Moss, Ralph W. *Complementary Oncology*. New York, NY: Thieme Medical Publishers, 2005.

Blaylock, Russell L. Excitotoxins: *The Taste that Kills*. Santa Fe, NM: Health Press, 1997.

Bloch, Abby S. (ed); Grant, Barbara (ed); Hamilton, Kathryn K. (ed); Thomson, Cynthia A. (ed). American Cancer Society Complete Guide to Nutrition for Cancer Survivors: *Eating Well, Staying Well During and After Cancer*. Atlanta, GA: American Cancer Society,2010.

Block, Keith; Weil, Andrew. *Life Over Cancer*. New York, NY: Bantam Books, 2009.

Boushey, Carol J.; Coulston, Ann M.; Rock, Cheryl L.; Monsen, Elaine. *Nutrition in the Prevention and Treatment of Disease*. Waltham, MA: Elsevier, 2001.

Brown, Susan E.; Trivieri, Jr., Larry. *The Acid Alkaline Food Guide.* Garden City Park, NY: Square One Publishers, 2006.

Campbell, T. Colin. *The China Study.* Dallas, TX: BenBella Books, Inc., 2006.

Carlson, Linda; Speca, Michael; Segal, Zindel. *Mindfulness-Based Cancer Recovery.* Oakland, CA: New Harbinger Publications, 2011.

Cordain, Loren. *The Paleo Diet.* New York, NY: John Wiley & Sons, Ltd., 2010.

Cragg, Gordon M. *Anticancer Agents from Natural Products.* Boca Raton, FL: CRC Press, 2005.

Cukier, Danie. *Coping With Chemotherapy and Radiation Therapy.* New York, NY: McGraw-Hill, 2004.

Dispenza, Joseph. *Live Better Longer.* San Francisco, CA: Harper San Francisco, 1997.

Fleishman, Stewart. *Learn to Live Through Cancer.* New York, NY: Demos Medical Publishing, 2011

Fuhrman, Joel. *Super Immunity.* New York, NY: HarperCollins, 2011.

Gershwin, M. E. *Spirulina in Human Nutrition and Health.* New York, NY: Taylor & Francis, 2007.

Gittleman, Ann Louise. *Get the Sugar Out,* Revised and Updated 2nd Edition. New York, NY: Crown Publishing Group, 2008.

Gorter, Robert; Peper, Erik. *Fighting Cancer.* Berkeley, CA: North Atlantic Books, 2011.

Grimes, Karlyn. *The Everything Anti-Inflammation Diet Book.* Cincinnati, Ohio: F+W Media, 2011.

Grossinger, Richard. *Planet Medicine.* Berkeley, CA: North Atlantic Books, 1995.

Hass, Elson. *Staying Healthy with Nutrition*. Berkeley, CA: Celestial Arts, 1992.

Hatherill, Robert J. *Eat to Beat Cancer*. Los Angeles, CA: Renaissance Books, 1998.

Hess, David J. *Can Bacteria Cause Cancer?* New York, NY: NYU Press, 1997.

Hoffer, Abram. *Orthomolecular Medicine for Everyone: Megavitamin Therapeutics for Families and Physicians*. Laguna Beach, CA: Basic Health Publications, 2008.

Irving, David Gerow. *The Protein Myth*. Ropley Hampshire: O-Books, 2011.

Jubb, Annie Padden; Jubb, David. *Secrets of an Alkaline Body*. Berkeley, CA: North Atlantic Books, 2012.

Kaelin, Carolyn M.; Coltrera, Francesca. *Living Through Breast Cancer*. New York, NY: McGraw-Hill, 2005.

Katsilambros, Nikolaos; Dimosthenopoulos, Charilaos; Kontogianni, Meropi D.; Manglara, Evangelia; Poulia, Kalliopi-Anna. *Clinical Nutrition in Practice*. Hoboken, NJ: John Wiley & Sons, Ltd., 2010.

Katz, Rebecca; Edelson, Mat. *One Bite at a Time*, revised paper. Berkeley, CA: Ten Speed Press, 2011.

Katzin, Carolyn F. *The Everything Cancer-Fighting Cookbook*. Cincinnati, Ohio: F+W Media, 2010.

Kelder, Peter. *Ancient Secret of the Fountain of Youth*. New York, NY: Doubleday, 1998.

Kelloff, Gary J.; Hawk, Ernest T.; Sigman, Caroline C. *Cancer Chemoprevention*. New York, NY: Springer, 2008.

Kelly, Lorraine; Anita. *Lorraine Kelly's Nutrition Made Easy*. New York, NY: Ebury Publishing, 2012.

Khalsa, Dharma Singh. *Food As Medicine*. New York, NY: Simon & Schuster, 2010.

Kumar, Nagi B. Nutritional. *Management of Cancer Treatment Effects*. New York, NY: Springer, 2012.

Langerak, Alan D.; Dreisbach, Luke P. *Chemotherapy Regimens and Cancer Care*. Austin, TX: Landes Bioscience, 2001.

Margel, Douglas L. *The Nutrient Dense Eating Plan*. Sydney: ReadHowYouWant, 2005.

McKay, Judith; Schacher, Tammy. *The Chemotherapy Survival Guide*. Oakland, CA: New Harbinger Publications, 2009.

Miller, Emmett E. Deep Healing: *The Essence of Mind/Body Medicine*. Carlsbad, CA: Hay House, 1997.

Minev, Boris R. *Cancer Management in Man*. New York, NY: Springer, 2011.

Missailidis, Sotiris. *Anticancer Therapeutics*. Hoboken, NJ: John Wiley & Sons, Ltd., 2008.

Mondoa, Emil I. *Sugars That Heal*. New York, NY: Random House Publishing Group, 2008.

Mowrey, Daniel B. *The Scientific Validation of Herbal Medicine*. Los Angeles, CA: Keats Publishing, 1986.

Mukherjee, Siddhartha. *The Emperor of All Maladies*. New York, NY: Simon & Schuster, 2010.

Mutanen, Marja; Pajari, Anne-Maria. *Vegetables Whole Grains, and Their Derivatives in Cancer Prevention*. New York, NY: Springer, 2011.

Newton, Herbert B. *Handbook of Brain Tumor Chemotherapy*. Waltham, MA: Elsevier, 2005.

Nicolle, Lorraine; Beirne, Ann Woodriff; Ash, Michael. *Biochemical Im-*

balances in Disease. Philadelphia, PA: Jessica Kingsley Publishers, 2010.

Ottoboni, Fred; Ottoboni, Alice. *The Modern Nutritional Diseases and How to Present Them*. Sparks, NV: Vincente Books, Inc., 2002.

Physicians Committee for Responsible Medicine. *Healthy Eating for Life to Prevent and Treat Cancer*. Hoboken, NJ: John Wiley & Sons, 2002.

Preedy, Victor R.; Watson, Ronald Ross. *Olives and Olive Oil in Health and Disease Prevention*. Waltham, MA: Elsevier, 2010.

Priestman, Terry. *Cancer Chemotherapy in Clinical Practice*. New York, NY: Springer, 2008.

Quillin, Patrick. *Beating Cancer with Nutrition*. Tulsa, OK: Nutrition Times Press, 2005.

Raffa, Robert B.; Tallarida, Ronald J. *Chemo Fog*. New York, NY: Springer, 2010.

Reid, Daniel. *The Tao Of Health, Sex and Longevity*. New York, NY: Simon & Schuster, 2011.

Rencun, Yu; Hai, Hong. *Cancer Management with Chinese Medicine*. Hackensack, NJ: World Scientific, 2012.

Ronzio, Robert. *The Encyclopedia of Nutrition and Good Health*. New York, NY: Infobase Publishing, 2003.

Salter, Andrew; Wiseman, Helen; Tucker, Gregory. *Phytonutrients*. New York, NY: John Wiley & Sons, Ltd., 2012.

Schwartz, Anna L.; Armstrong, Lance. *Cancer Fitness*. Simon & Schuster, 2004.

Seeram, Navindra P.; Stoner, Gary D. *Berries and Cancer Prevention*. New York, NY: Springer, 2011.

Servan-Schreiber, David. *Anticancer, A New Way of Life*. New York, NY: Viking Adult, 2009.

Shaw, Clare. *Nutrition and Cancer*. Hoboken, NJ: John Wiley & Sons, Ltd., 2010.

Silver, Julie. *You Can Heal Yourself*. New York, NY: St. Martin's Paperbacks, 2012.

Silverman, Dan; Davidson, Idelle. *Your Brain After Chemo*. Cambridge, MA: Da Capo Press, 2009.

Slaga, Thomas J.; Keuneke, Robin. *The Detox Revolution*. New York, NY: McGraw-Hill, 2003.

Somers, Suzanne. *Knockout*. New York, NY: Crown Publishing Group, 2009.

Thomas, Gareth. *Fundamentals of Medicinal Chemistry*. Hoboken, NJ: John Wiley & Sons, Ltd., 2004.

Thompson, Jennifer Trainer. *Very Blueberry*. Berkeley, CA: Ten Speed Press, 2011.

Tierra, Michael. *The Way of Herbs*. New York, NY: Pocket Books, 1980.

Tyson, Richard. Rich Remedies: *My Amazing Natural Self-Healing Discoveries*. Bloomington, IN: iUniverse, 2008.

Visel, Dave. *Living with Cancer*. New Brunswick, NJ: Rutgers University Press, 2006.

Watson, Ronald Ross. *Functional Foods and Nutraceuticals in Cancer Prevention*. Hoboken, NJ: John Wiley & Sons, Ltd., 2008.

Weihofen, Donna L.; Robbins, JoAnne; Sullivan, Paula A. *Easy-to-Swallow, Easy-to-Chew Cookbook*. Hoboken, NJ: John Wiley & Sons, Ltd., 2002.

Weil, Andrew. *Health and Healing*. New York, NY: Houghton Mifflin Company, 1983.

Williams-Huw, Michelle. *My Mummy Wears a Wig—Does Yours?* Mid Glamorgan: Accent Press Ltd., 2007.

Wolff, Meg. *A Life in Balance.* Camden ME: Down East Books, 2010.

Wood, Matthew. Vitalism: *The History of Herbalism, Homeopathy, and Flower Essences.* Berkeley, CA: North Atlantic Books, 1992.

World Health Organization. *Nutrition and the Prevention of Chronic Diseases.* Geneva: World Health Organization, 2003.

Index

STAY HEALTHY DURING CHEMO

C

D

E

F

To Our Readers

Conari Press, an imprint of Red Wheel/Weiser, publishes books on topics ranging from spirituality, personal growth, and relationships to women's issues, parenting, and social issues. Our mission is to publish quality books that will make a difference in people's lives— how we feel about ourselves and how we relate to one another. We value integrity, compassion, and receptivity, both in the books we publish and in the way we do business.

Our readers are our most important resource, and we appreciate your input, suggestions, and ideas about what you would like to see published.

Visit our website at www.redwheelweiser.com to learn about our upcoming books and free downloads, and be sure to go to www. redwheelweiser.com/newsletter/ to sign up for newsletters and exclusive offers.

You can also contact us at info@rwwbooks.com.

Conari Press
an imprint of Red Wheel/Weiser, LLC
65 Parker Street, Suite 7
Newburyport, MA 01950